D0125063

WHAT EVERY
PARENT
SHOULD KNOW ABOUT
VACCINES

PAUL A. OFFIT, M.D.

LOUIS M. BELL, M.D.

Macmillan • USA

This publication contains the opinions and ideas of its authors. It is intended to provide helpful and informative material on the subject matter covered. It is sold with the understanding that the authors and publisher are not engaged in rendering medical or other professional services in this book. If the reader requires personal medical or health assistance or advice, a competent professional should be consulted.

The authors and publisher specifically disclaim any responsibility for any liability, loss, or risk, personal or otherwise, which is incurred as a consequence, directly or indirectly, of the use and application of any of the contents of this book.

MACMILLAN
A Simon & Schuster Macmillan Company
1633 Broadway
New York, NY 10019-6785

Macmillan Publishing books may be purchased for business or sales promotional use. For information please write: Special Markets Department, Macmillan Publishing USA, 1633 Broadway, New York, NY 10019-6785.

Library of Congress Cataloging-in-Publication Data

Offit, Paul A.
    What every parent should know about vaccines / Paul A. Offit, Louis M. Bell.
        p.   cm.
    Includes bibliographical references and index.
    ISBN 0-02-862009-7 (pbk.: alk. paper)
    1. Vaccination of children—Popular works. 2. Vaccines. I. Bell,
Louis M. II. Title.
RJ240.039   1998
97-31780
615'.372'083—dc21
    CIP

Printed in the United States of America

10 9 8 7 6 5 4 3 2 1

For Bonnie, Will, and Emily
and Barbara, Susan, Amy, Christopher, and Sarah
with all our love

*Those who cannot remember the past are condemned
to repeat it.*
George Santayana (1863–1952)
From "The Life of Reason" (1905)

*In the face of such diseases, the most dangerous
experiment of all is to do nothing.*
Joseph Stokes, Jr., MD (1896–1972)
From **The New England Journal of Medicine,** *1967,
in reference to the deaths caused by measles and
mumps viruses*

Acknowledgments

The authors wish to acknowledge the physicians, scientists, mothers, fathers, and friends whose knowledge of vaccines and commitment to children helped to shape this book: Jani Bergan; Shirley Bonnem; Candace Chacona; Christina Chan, MD; H. Fred Clark, PhD; David Cobb; Susan Coffin, MD; Charles deTaisne, PhD; R. Gordon Douglas, MD; Joseph Eiden, MD, PhD; Ronald Ellis, PhD; Bonnie Fass-Offit, MD; Denise Freeman; Richard Gesser, MD; Beth Hibbs, RN, MPH; Maurice Hilleman, PhD; Jacqueline Jenkins; Jennifer Lloyd, MD; Lois and Phillip Macht; Peggy McGratty; Charlotte Moser; Deborah Goodman Naisch; Mindy and Carl Offit; Peter Paradiso, PhD; Larry Pickering, MD; Stanley Plotkin, MD; Geoffrey Porges, MBBS; Bob Ruffner; Jerald Sadoff, MD; Allan Shaw, PhD; Stuart Starr, MD; Gina Terracino, MD; Judith Thalheimer, MD; Thomas Vernon, MD; Barbara Watson, MD; Jeffrey Weiser, MD; Deborah Wexler, MD; Amy Wilen; Susan Wei Winnick, and John Zimmerman.

In addition, we wish to thank Joline Fontaine, Nancy Love, and Betsy Thorpe for their unswerving belief in this project.

CONTENTS

INTRODUCTION

Almost every child in this country gets vaccinations, and therefore almost every parent has questions about them. Parents want to know what vaccines are made of, if they work, and whether they are safe. They want to know why there are so many shots and whether they are all really necessary. Mostly, they want to know what their children are getting when they have these shots.

With a new vaccine on the market (chickenpox), a debate among physicians about whether we should still use an old vaccine (oral polio), and an improved component of a vaccine that rarely caused serious side effects (whooping cough or pertussis), parents have a lot of questions for their doctors.

Recently a law was passed that requires doctors to explain the risks and benefits of vaccines before getting permission from parents to use them. Unfortunately, doctors, often restricted by a busy schedule, may not have enough time to answer all the parents' questions.

The purpose of this book is to help answer the questions parents have about vaccines. We'll explain what vaccines are made of, how they are made, how they work, and the risks associated with them. We'll describe the diseases that vaccines protect against and why it's still important to build defenses against them.

We hope this book will help parents wade through the misinformation that is occasionally offered by newspapers, television programs, and well-meaning friends and family. More importantly, we hope that this book will help parents make the choices that are best for their children.

PART ONE

WHAT ARE VACCINES?

C H A P T E R 1

DO WE STILL NEED VACCINES?

Vaccines are medicine's bright and shining stars. Before vaccines, parents in the United States could expect that every year:

- *Polio would paralyze 10,000 children.*
- *Rubella ("German measles") would cause birth defects and mental retardation in as many as 20,000 newborns.*
- *Measles would infect about 4 million children, killing 3,000.*
- *Diphtheria would be one of the most common causes of death in school-aged children.*
- *A bacterium called Hib would cause meningitis in 25,000 children, leaving many with permanent brain damage.*
- *Pertussis ("whooping cough") would kill 8,000 children, most of whom were less than 1 year of age.*

Vaccines have changed those horrifying numbers. Now parents can expect that every year in the United States there will be only about two cases of diphtheria, three cases of birth defects from rubella, and no cases of polio. Children have benefited more from vaccines than from any other preventive program in history (with the possible exception of the purification of drinking water).

However, because vaccines have almost eliminated certain infections, some parents are reexamining their usefulness. Do we still need vaccines? Do their benefits still outweigh their risks? As you will see in the pages that follow, the answers to both of these questions is yes. Unfortunately, the viral and bacterial diseases that are preventable by vaccines either continue to infect children in this country or are only a plane ride away from causing an outbreak.

CHAPTER 2

HOW DO VACCINES WORK?

Ed and Emily are both 5 years old. Emily got a measles vaccine when she was 15 months old. She had soreness and tenderness for two days where the shot was given. Ed never got the vaccine.

One day both Ed and Emily were exposed in their classroom to a third child, who had measles and who was very contagious.

About one week later Ed got the measles. He had a cough, runny nose, and "pink eye." Two days after that he got a rash that started on his face and spread to the rest of his body. He had a fever of 104°F and started to have difficulty breathing. His doctor requested a chest X ray and found that Ed had pneumonia (not at all uncommon with measles). After having to spend about a week in the hospital, Ed, fortunately, got better.

Emily never caught the measles to which she was exposed.

5

Because Ed caught the measles, he will never get measles again. Because Emily got the measles vaccine, she will never get measles. They are both now immune to measles.

But Ed paid a high price for his immunity. He was very sick for over a week. Emily only had a sore arm.

How did Emily get immunity without first getting sick?

First we need to understand what happened to Ed and Emily.

WHAT HAPPENED TO ED

Ed caught measles from another child with measles who was coughing. When the child coughed, thousands of tiny droplets were sprayed into the air near Ed's mouth. Inside many of these droplets were hundreds of measles viruses.

Once the measles viruses entered Ed's body, their mission was clear: to make copies of themselves (or replicate) over and over again. The measles viruses replicated in Ed's skin and lungs, causing Ed's symptoms of rash and pneumonia. By the time the replication process was finished, hundreds of measles viruses had become billions of measles viruses.

While Ed was infected with measles, his body produced antibodies to the virus. Antibodies are proteins that are made by B cells in the blood and lymph nodes. These antibodies against measles virus in part helped Ed eliminate the virus from his body. The B cells that made antibodies to measles virus will probably hang around in Ed's body for the rest of his life as memory B cells. The next time Ed is exposed to measles, these memory B cells will make antibodies that will kill (or neutralize) the measles virus before it can make him sick. Because Ed now has memory B cells specific for measles virus, he is said to be immune to measles.

What Happened to Emily

The measles virus that Emily was given in the vaccine when she was a toddler was very different from the one that Ed caught. Emily was given a measles virus that was weakened so that it couldn't replicate very well. Because it replicated poorly, it didn't make Emily sick.

But the weakened version of measles that Emily was given still caused her to produce antibodies against measles and develop memory B cells that she will probably have for the rest of her life. When Emily was exposed to the measles virus in her classroom, these memory B cells made antibodies that killed the virus before it could make her sick. Therefore, because of the vaccine, Emily was also immune to measles.

How Viruses and Bacteria Make You Sick

What happened to Emily is what happens to children when they get a vaccine: They get immunity without getting sick. To know how vaccines do this, we need to understand how viruses and bacteria make you sick.

Viruses and bacteria are like M & Ms.

M & Ms are shells that contain chocolate centers. Viruses and bacteria are shells that contain substances called genes. The genes are simply blueprints that tell the viruses and bacteria how to make copies of themselves, or replicate.

One virus can make hundreds of copies of itself in as little as 8 to 12 hours, and each newly created virus can do the same. It is easy to see how the hundreds of viruses to which Ed was exposed could become billions of viruses within one week.

Many bacteria make you sick just the way viruses do: by causing damage in places where the bacteria are replicating. Some bacteria make you sick by manufacturing a harmful protein called toxin. In this case it is the toxin, not the bacteria, that does the damage.

Ed and Emily had different experiences because they were exposed to different measles viruses. The measles virus Ed caught from another child (the so-called wild-type virus) replicated to billions of viruses that caused damage to his skin and lungs. The weakened measles virus Emily was given as a shot (the vaccine virus) probably replicated to form only hundreds of viruses. This isn't very much replication, so Emily didn't get sick. But Emily's body had "seen" enough measles to develop immunity.

To summarize how vaccines work:

- Viruses and bacteria cause disease by replicating well inside the body and thus damaging cells such as those in the skin and lungs.

- The viruses and bacteria in vaccines don't replicate well or don't replicate at all.

- Therefore, vaccines don't cause the diseases that are usually caused by viruses and bacteria.

- A child given a vaccine is exposed to just enough of the virus or bacteria to cause immunity (memory B cells).

- Memory B cells produce the antibodies needed to destroy viruses and bacteria before they make you sick. These cells often last a lifetime.

CHAPTER 3

HOW ARE
VACCINES
MADE?

Vaccines are made by taking viruses or bacteria and weakening them so that they can't replicate (or divide) very well or so that they can't replicate at all. Children given vaccines are exposed to enough of the virus or bacteria to develop immunity, but not enough to make them sick. There are four ways that viruses and bacteria are weakened to make vaccines:

1. **Change the virus blueprint (or genes) so that the virus replicates poorly.** This is how the measles, mumps, rubella, varicella, and oral polio vaccines are made.

    The virus blueprint is changed by a technique called cell-culture adaptation (see below). Because viruses can still to some extent make copies of themselves after cell culture-adaptation (and therefore are still alive), they are often referred to as live, attenuated (or weakened) viruses.

9

How Measles Viruses Are Weakened to Make a Vaccine

Measles viruses normally grow in cells that line the back of a child's throat and in cells lining the lung. The measles vaccine was made by taking measles virus from the throat of an infected child (the "wild-type" virus) and adapting it to growth in specialized cells grown in the laboratory (a process called cell-culture adaptation). As the virus becomes better and better able to grow in these specialized cells, it becomes less and less able to grow in a child's skin or lungs. When this cell-culture adapted virus (or vaccine virus) is given to a child, it replicates only a little before it is eliminated from the body.

2. **Destroy the virus blueprint (or genes) so that the virus can't replicate at all.** This is how the "killed" polio vaccine (or polio shot) is made. Vaccine virus is made by treating polio virus with the chemical formaldehyde. This treatment permanently destroys the polio genes so that the virus can no longer replicate.

3. **Use only a part of the virus or bacteria.** This is how the Hib, hepatitis B, and (in part) pertussis vaccines are made. Because the viral or bacterial genes are not present in the vaccine, the viruses or bacteria can't replicate.

4. **Take the toxin that is released from the bacteria, purify it, and kill it so it can't do any harm.** Some bacteria cause disease not by replicating but by manufacturing harmful proteins called toxins. For example, bacteria like diphtheria, tetanus, and pertussis (whooping cough) all cause disease by producing toxins. To make vaccines against these bacteria, toxins are purified and killed with chemicals (such as formaldehyde). Again, because bacterial genes are not part of the vaccine, bacteria can't replicate.

Some Vaccines Are Like Sparring Partners . . .

Most children infected with viruses survive without any problems. These children fought and won the big fight against those infections without being permanently harmed by them. However, not all children are as lucky.

Live, weakened viral vaccines are like sparring partners getting children ready for a fight. Sparring partners engage fighters in a little fight (without hurting them) to prepare them for a big one.

Children immunized with live, weakened viral vaccines (such as measles, mumps, rubella, chickenpox, and polio) are actually infected with a weakened form of the real virus. This weakened form spars with the child and helps cause immunity without harming the child. When it's time for the big fight (meaning the child is exposed to the natural or "wild-type" virus), the child is ready and able for the match and wins hands-down.

. . . And Others Are Like Vitamin C

Protective immunity against a particular virus or bacteria is often directed against one part of that virus or bacteria. Vaccines that use part of the shell of the virus or bacteria (such as hepatitis B or Hib) or those that use an inactivated toxin (such as pertussis, diphtheria, and tetanus) are examples of immunizations using the critical part of a virus or bacteria.

Many people drink orange juice for the vitamin C. Some people take the essence of the orange juice by taking purified vitamin C. This is analogous to vaccine strategies that use the essence of the virus or bacteria necessary for protection. In both cases the purified, final product is made from natural ingredients.

WHY AREN'T ALL VACCINES MADE THE SAME WAY?

Wouldn't it be easier just to use the same strategy to make all vaccines?

There are many reasons why different vaccine strategies are used for different infections. For example, both measles and hepatitis B are viruses. The measles vaccine was made by weakening the virus by cell-culture adaptation, as discussed above. However, it is very difficult to grow hepatitis B virus in cells, so the process of cell-culture adaptation couldn't be easily used to make a hepatitis B virus vaccine. Also, the protective immune response against hepatitis B virus is directed for the most part against just one protein on the surface of the virus (which is not true for measles virus). Therefore, a vaccine for hepatitis B virus was made using just that one hepatitis B virus protein.

HOW VACCINES ARE ACTUALLY MADE (THE STORY OF THE MUMPS VACCINE)

On March 30, 1963, Jeryl Lynn Hilleman, the 5-year-old daughter of Maurice Hilleman, said to her father, "Daddy, my neck hurts!" It was 1:00 A.M. Maurice Hilleman, PhD, picked up his daughter, carefully examined her throat and neck, and thought to himself, "Oh my God, she has the mumps." Dr. Hilleman's next move was unusual. He went to his research laboratory, picked up some cotton swabs and several tubes of broth (a nutrient-rich fluid in which viruses are kept alive), and brought them home. He then went back up to Jeryl Lynn's room, woke her up, swabbed the back of her throat, placed the swab in the broth, and went back to his laboratory.

In 1963 mumps was a highly prevalent and highly contagious disease in the United States. Most people knew mumps as a painful swelling of the salivary glands (the parotid glands), which are located just below the ear. However, mumps virus also caused a number of other serious problems. For example, mumps virus infected the brain, causing encephalitis, or lining of the brain, causing meningitis, in about half of all children that were infected. As a result, mumps virus was one of the most common causes of acquired (as distinct from congenital) deafness in children. Mumps virus also infected the pancreas, the organ that makes insulin, occasionally resulting in severe diabetes. Dr. Hilleman, at the time the director of Virus and Cell Biology Research at Merck, Sharpe and Dohme Laboratories, desperately wanted to make a vaccine to prevent these serious complications.

Despite Dr. Hilleman's considerable understanding of viruses and how they worked, he needed help to develop the mumps vaccine. This help came from his daughter the night she came down with the mumps. Dr. Hilleman needed to find a strain of mumps virus that *couldn't* infect the lining of the brain or the brain itself, and, fortunately, this was exactly the kind of strain that infected Jeryl Lynn. Now that more than 300 million doses of the "Jeryl Lynn" strain of mumps vaccine have been given to children throughout the world, the serious complications of mumps infection have been virtually eliminated from most countries.

So just how did Dr. Hilleman get the virus that made his daughter sick to protect other children from this occasionally serious disease?

In the early morning hours of March 30, 1963, Dr. Hilleman took the virus that he had obtained from the back of Jeryl Lynn's throat and inoculated it into hen's eggs. Dr. Hilleman wanted the mumps virus taken from Jeryl Lynn to grow in the cells that were part of the chick embryo. After several days, he removed fluid from the center of the eggs and inoculated this fluid into other hen's eggs. This process was done 12 times. The purpose of growing the virus repeatedly (or in serial passage) in hen's eggs was to weaken it. As the virus became better and better able to grow in hen's eggs it became less and less able to grow in children due to cell-culture adaptation (discussed above). Dr. Hilleman wanted the virus to grow well enough in children so that they developed immunity, but not so well that they would get sick as a result.

After passaging the virus 12 times in hen's eggs (called level A virus), Dr. Hilleman took some of the virus and grew it five more times in chick embryo cells that were grown in laboratory flasks (level B virus). Next, the level A and B viruses were tested to make sure that there were no other viruses, bacteria, or fungi contaminating the vaccine. The viruses were then tested for safety in experimental animals. When the mumps viruses from levels A and B were shown to be safe in experimental animals and free from other infectious agents, they were approved for further testing in children by the U.S. Bureau of Biologics. Two years had now elapsed since Dr. Hilleman first isolated the mumps virus from his daughter.

The year was 1965, and it was time to test the mumps viruses from levels A and B in children. To do this, Dr. Hilleman called on his friends and coworkers Drs. Joseph Stokes, Jr., and Robert Weibel, both professors in pediatrics at The University of Pennsylvania School of Medicine and at The Children's Hospital of Philadelphia. Their first challenge was to make sure that the mumps viruses were safe in children. About 30 children per group were injected into the arm with the vaccines from level A or B. Both levels A and B induced mumps virus-specific antibodies in the blood, but whereas level A vaccine still caused mild swelling and tenderness of the salivary glands in some children, level B did not. So level B vaccine was determined to be safe. The next step was to find out whether it could protect children against the mumps.

Drs. Stokes and Weibel went to civic groups and churches in the Havertown-Springfield area of Philadelphia and recruited about 6,300 children who had never before been exposed to mumps virus. These children were injected with level B vaccine, and the investigators waited for a natural outbreak of mumps virus to occur. The results were dramatic: 97 percent of inoculated children developed antibodies to the vaccine, and 97 percent were protected when an outbreak of mumps swept through their community. The vaccine was licensed by the Federal Regulatory Agency (now the FDA) in December of 1967, only four years after Jeryl Lynn Hilleman was infected with mumps. One of the first recipients of the new vaccine was Jeryl Lynn's younger sister, Kirsten.

The mumps vaccine that is administered to children today in combination with vaccines against measles and rubella (see Chapter 10) is identical to the vaccine that was used in 1967.

HARD LESSONS ON THE VACCINE ROAD

There are currently ten recommended vaccines for use in all children. All ten have a remarkable record of safety and efficacy. However, the development of successful vaccines is not always as linear and unburdened as that of the mumps vaccine. There have been, on occasion, hard lessons. Two instructive cases are detailed below:

THE CUTTER INCIDENT

Probably the most disastrous event in the history of vaccine making occurred in 1955. The event was chronicled in 1963 in a now classic article in the *American Journal of Hygiene* by Drs. Neal Nathanson and Alexander Langmuir. The first paragraph of that article is shown below:

> *On April 25, 1955, an infant with paralytic poliomyelitis was admitted to Michael Reese Hospital, Chicago, Illinois. The patient had been inoculated in the buttock with Cutter vaccine on April 16, and developed flaccid [complete] paralysis of both legs on April 24. The case was reported by the Chicago Board of Health to the Public Health Service on April 25. On April 26 the California State Health Department reported 5 more cases of paralytic poliomyelitis in Cutter vaccinees. All developed within 4 to 10 days of vaccination and all had paralytic involvement of the inoculated arm. This was the beginning of the Cutter incident.*

In mid-1950s America, polio was a common and feared disease. Every year about 15,000 people (most of them children) were paralyzed or killed by this virus. The first vaccine to meet this challenge was that developed by Dr. Jonas Salk. Dr. Salk theorized that if you took poliovirus, killed it with formaldehyde, and injected it into the muscles, you could protect children and adults from paralytic poliovirus. Dr. Salk's theory was proven correct by Thomas Francis in field trials performed between 1954 and 1955—trials in which about 200,000 children were immunized. On April 12, 1955 (ten years to the day after the death of one of polio's most famous victims, Franklin Delano Roosevelt), the announcement of the success of the polio vaccine made front-page headlines across the country. Six companies were licensed to produce and distribute this "killed" or inactivated polio vaccine. One of those companies was Cutter Laboratories.

In mid-April 1955, about 400,000 people (most of them first and second graders) were immunized with the polio vaccine made by Cutter Laboratories. Over the two months that followed, 94 cases of paralysis occurred among those vaccinated, 126 cases among contacts living in the home of those vaccinated, and 140 cases among community contacts. Drs. Nathanson and Langmuir proved that these cases were the result of receiving the Cutter vaccine.

How could this happen? Like the measles vaccine described above, the poliovirus used to make poliovirus vaccine was grown in cells in the laboratory. In the case of Cutter Laboratories, clumps of these cells had formed and settled at the bottom of the flasks. The formaldehyde that was used to kill the virus was thus unable to penetrate into the center of all the clumps and effectively kill all the poliovirus. The result was that live, deadly poliovirus was given into the arms of some young children. The fact that there was a problem with the vaccine was made obvious in that vaccinated children often developed paralysis in the arm that was inoculated (usually poliovirus causes paralysis in the legs).

The result of this disaster was that more stringent guidelines for the manufacture and testing of poliovirus vaccine were put in place by what is now the Food and Drug Administration. Over the 30 years since the Cutter incident, there has not been one case of paralysis in a child receiving the "killed" vaccine, and the paralysis and death caused by natural poliovirus has been eliminated from the United States. The current safety tests required for licensure of poliovirus vaccines insure that the Cutter incident will never happen again.

THE STORY OF THE RSV VACCINE

Respiratory Syncytial Virus, or RSV, is a virus that infects the lungs of young children, usually those less than 2 years old. RSV is one of the biggest killers of infants and young children in the United States: 80,000 children are hospitalized and between 4,000 and 5,000 die each year, usually because of severe pneumonia (see Chapter 27 for more details).

Because of the importance of RSV, there has been a great deal of interest in preventing the disease with an effective vaccine. However, early attempts to develop an RSV vaccine were frustrated by some surprising results.

In the mid-1960s, a number of investigators were trying to make a successful RSV vaccine. The most common approach at the time was to take RSV and inactivate it with formaldehyde. The vaccine was given in the muscles of first adults and then children to make sure that it was safe. Once the vaccine was found to be safe, infants and young children were immunized to see whether the vaccine protected them against the pneumonia caused by RSV.

Every year outbreaks of RSV sweep across the country, so after the children were immunized the investigators only had to wait for one of these natural outbreaks to occur. What they found took them by surprise. Not only were children not protected against RSV, but after natural infection those who were immunized developed more severe pneumonia than those who weren't. Some of those who were immunized and later became infected with RSV had to be admitted to the hospital and artificially ventilated.

The strategy used by these investigators (specifically, to take whole, live RSV and kill it with formaldehyde) had been used prior to 1960 to make successful vaccines against influenza, polio, and rabies, and has since been used to make successful vaccines against hepatitis A virus. The reasons for the failure of the inactivated RSV vaccine remain somewhat unclear.

Because the initial field trials showed that the vaccine didn't work, the RSV vaccine was never licensed or manufactured. It was back to the drawing boards. Although we still don't have an RSV vaccine, recent trials in children have shown some promise.

CHAPTER 4

ARE VACCINES SAFE?

Whether we realize it or not, we're all gamblers in everyday life. There are risks in even the most routine activities:

- *We take a bath, even though every year in the United States about 350 people are killed in bath-related accidents.*
- *We eat breakfast, even though every year about 200 people are killed when food lodges in their windpipe.*
- *We walk outside on a rainy day, even though every year about 100 people are struck and killed by lightning.*

We do these things because we think that the odds are heavily in our favor. We are willing to take small risks to enjoy large benefits. If we wanted, we could avoid many of these risks by simply staying in our home, living in a protective bubble, eating carefully prepared soft foods, and having armed guards at our door. However, few people are willing to do this.

But of course there are other risks that are easier to lessen. Every day we are at risk of catching viral or bacterial infections. For many types of infections the risks are actually quite high. For example, it is estimated that children less than 6 years old will have an average of six to eight infections every year. This is where vaccines come in. Vaccines are examples of taking small risks (side effects from the vaccine) to enjoy large benefits (avoidance of permanent disabilities or death caused by infection).

The question for vaccines is, "Do the benefits outweigh the risks?" There is probably no better way to answer this question than to tell the story of the vaccine with the highest rate of side effects, pertussis (better known as whooping cough).

THE PERTUSSIS STORY

The pertussis vaccine was first developed in the mid-1940s. It soon became clear that this vaccine had significant side effects. The side effects from the original pertussis vaccine, the one used in the formulation called DTP (which stands for *D*iphtheria, *T*etanus, *P*ertussis), are shown below:

Mild side effects	*Number of side effects per number of doses given*
Pain where the shot was given	1 per 2 doses
Swelling where the shot was given	2 per 5 doses
Fever of 100.4°F or greater	1 per 2 doses
Fretfulness	1 per 2 doses
Drowsiness	1 per 3 doses
Vomiting	1 per 15 doses

Severe side effects	*Number of side effects per number of doses given*
Persistent, inconsolable crying (for more than 3 hours)	1 per 100 doses
Fever of 105°F or greater	1 per 330 doses
Seizures	1 per 1,750 doses

Because the risk of side effects with the old pertussis vaccine was high, some parents chose not to vaccinate their children. Was this the right choice? Or, asked another way, were children at greater risk from the vaccine or the disease? To answer these questions we need only look at what happened to children in Japan in the late 1970s.

In 1975, the Japanese Ministry of Health and Welfare, in response to negative publicity on the pertussis vaccine, imposed a moratorium on its use. In the three years before the moratorium, there were 400 cases of pertussis and 10 associated deaths. In the three years following discontinuation of the vaccine, there were 13,000 cases of pertussis and 113 associated deaths. It should be noted that although the side effects from the original pertussis vaccine were high, no child ever died from pertussis vaccine. The children of Japan proved in a clear and definitive way that the benefits of receiving the vaccine far outweighed the risks.

Today, parents have an easier choice about the pertussis vaccine, because a new one with fewer side effects for infants, first made available in the fall of 1996, is now available for use in all children (see Chapter 7).

THE NATIONAL VACCINE INJURY COMPENSATION PROGRAM

Unfortunately, the pertussis vaccine story didn't end with the lessons from Japan. In 1974, physicians working at The Hospital for Sick Children in London reported 36 children thought to suffer from a variety of neurological disorders following receipt of the DTP vaccine. In response to this report, a study was performed in England to determine whether the DTP vaccine caused permanent brain damage. The study was called the National Childhood Encephalopathy Study (encephalopathy means disease of the brain), or NCES. Data from this study were interpreted as showing that the DTP vaccine caused one case of permanent brain damage for every 310,000 doses of DTP given.

The report from England that DTP caused permanent brain damage in children was destructive for two reasons. First, it was wrong. A review of the NCES study by the Institute of Medicine (an independent research organization in the United States chartered by the National Academy of Sciences) showed that the DTP vaccine *didn't* cause permanent brain damage. Second, American lawyers, taking advantage of the fear and misinformation surrounding the vaccine, unleashed a flood of lawsuits claiming that it not only caused permanent brain damage but also caused unexplained coma, epilepsy, and sudden infant death syndrome (SIDS). The burden of defending these lawsuits prompted many vaccine makers to stop manufacturing the pertussis vaccine, and soon there were severe shortages. Because of these shortages, the United States was poised to repeat the mistake made by Japan a decade earlier.

Fortunately, the crisis was averted. In 1986, a collaborative effort between the American Academy of Pediatrics, vaccine makers, parents, and lawyers created the National Vaccine Compensation Act (Public Law 99-660). The cornerstone of this act was the National Vaccine Injury Compensation Program (NVICP). This program, funded by a federal excise tax on all vaccines, compensated those with vaccine-related injuries and to some extent protected vaccine makers from lawsuits.

How did the NVICP decide what constituted a "vaccine-related injury"? Unfortunately, there wasn't much help from published studies, so the NVICP took their best guess. They constructed a Vaccine Injury Table that included side effects a group made up of scientists, physicians, parents, and lawyers felt were most likely to be associated with vaccines. Compensation by this program was based on a "legal presumption of causation" even if there was no medical evidence showing causation.

Because of the NVICP, the crisis was ended. Vaccine litigation in court dramatically declined from a peak of 255 claims in 1986 to 20 claims in 1993. As a result, vaccine prices stabilized, and vaccine makers in this country not only continued to make existing vaccines, but increased expenditures on the research and development of new ones.

THE INSTITUTE OF MEDICINE STUDIES

Probably the most important legacy of the NVICP was a law mandating a careful review of potential side effects caused by vaccines. These studies were performed by the Institute of Medicine and now form the basis of our understanding about what side effects can be caused by vaccines. The Institute of Medicine studied the side effects caused by pertussis, rubella, measles, mumps, diphtheria, tetanus, polio, hepatitis B, and haemophilus influenzae type B vaccines; reports of these studies were released in 1991 and 1994.

The Institute of Medicine determined whether vaccines caused serious side effects by doing the following:

- Employing 31 electronic databases to identify about 2,000 relevant citations.

- Reviewing 550 unpublished case reports. Most of these reports came from a passive surveillance system under the supervision of the Centers for Disease Control and Prevention. Many of the reports came from private citizens.

- Allowing all private citizens to express their concerns about vaccines in four meetings that were open to the public.

The Institute of Medicine found that although vaccines can *definitely* cause serious side effects, these side effects are extremely rare. Their nature and frequency will be discussed in the chapters on individual vaccines.

"Seen" and "Unseen" Risks

We tend to overestimate the "seen" as compared with the "unseen" risks. For example, in 1989, CBS News's *60 Minutes* claimed that a pesticide used on apples (under the trade name Alar) could cause cancer in children. This story sparked a panic that resulted in the destruction of millions of dollars' worth of apples and apple products and the loss of farms for many apple growers (even those who didn't use Alar).

Man-made (or synthetic) toxins are a "seen" risk. We know we make them, we know we put them into the environment, and we know where we put them. But the "unseen" risks are actually much greater. For example, there are thousands of natural toxins in the environment. Plants make toxins to protect themselves from molds and plant-eating animals. Some of these toxins clearly cause cancer, and some are highly lethal. Even though trace amounts of these toxins are present in milk, corn, peanuts, and eggs, you almost never hear about them. Our diet contains about 10,000 times more natural toxins than synthetic ones.

The comparison between synthetic and natural toxins can also be made with vaccines and infections. Over the first five years of life, most children will receive ten different vaccines. Vaccines are a "seen" risk; we know who makes them, how they are made, and who gets them. But what are the "unseen" risks? Thousands of different kinds of potentially harmful viruses and bacteria are part of our daily environment. Many people would be surprised to know that you are more likely to acquire germs from the money in your pocket than from visiting a friend in the hospital. About half of all paper currency carries infectious organisms.

ARE VACCINES SAFE?

So the answer to the question "Are vaccines safe?" depends on how you define the word *safe*. If you define *safe* as completely free of any possible negative effects, then the answer is no. But nothing is completely safe (not even money).

The better question is "Do the benefits of vaccines (avoiding infections) outweigh their risks (side effects)?" To answer this question you need three pieces of information:

1. What are the chances of catching a particular infection?

2. What are the risks of side effects from a particular vaccine?

3. How effective is the vaccine in preventing disease?

As you will see in the sections that follow, the chances of permanent harm from vaccines are lower than those of being struck by lightning.

Chapter 5

WHO RECOMMENDS VACCINES?

Parents are told by doctors that vaccines are "recommended" and by schools that vaccines are "required." Few parents understand how these decisions are made and who makes them.

Three types of endorsement are usually in place before vaccines are given to children: approval, recommendation, and requirement. The agencies and considerations involved in each of these decisions are different.

APPROVAL

Before pharmaceutical companies test a vaccine in children, they must first obtain an Investigational New Drug license, or IND. Approval for this license is granted by the Food and Drug Administration, or FDA.

An IND license is awarded only if companies have shown that the vaccine is completely safe in animals and is not contaminated with other microorganisms not meant to be part of the vaccine, such as fungi, bacteria, or viruses.

Once an IND license is obtained, the manufacturer tests the vaccine in children to make sure it is safe and effective. This information is then submitted to the FDA for approval (or licensure) of the vaccine. FDA approval is based on two questions: "Is the vaccine *safe?*" and "Is the vaccine *effective?*" Therefore, the FDA is concerned solely with the risk–benefit ratio of the vaccine. Once this approval is obtained, the pharmaceutical company has the right to sell the vaccine.

RECOMMENDATION

Even after a vaccine has been approved by the FDA, doctors will usually wait until it is recommended before giving it to their patients. However, to our knowledge, there has never been a vaccine that was approved by the FDA and not recommended for use.

There are primarily two committees that recommend the use of vaccines for children: the Advisory Committee on Immunization Practices, or ACIP (part of the Centers for Disease Control and Prevention), and the Infectious Disease Committee of the American Academy of Pediatrics (AAP). Each of these advisory bodies is composed of 10 to 15 physicians and scientists with extensive experience in infectious diseases, immunology, and vaccine research. (Voting members of these committees are not allowed to have any financial connection to vaccine manufacturers.) The data considered by these agencies is broader than that considered by the FDA. Whereas the FDA considers only whether vaccines work and are safe, advisory bodies consider how much vaccines *cost* and how to best *use* them. In other words, the FDA considers only risk–benefit ratios, whereas advisory bodies also consider cost–benefit ratios.

Two recent stories show how advisory bodies consider the cost and use of vaccines.

The issue of vaccine *cost* is best shown by the chickenpox (or varicella) vaccine. Compared to diseases such as measles, mumps, and rubella, varicella is a relatively benign illness with only occasional serious consequences (see Chapter 12 for more information).

The varicella vaccine was licensed by the FDA in March of 1995. One of the questions that the advisory bodies asked when the vaccine was licensed was "What is the estimated cost–benefit ratio of the varicella vaccine?" In other words, what is the projected cost of immunizing all children in the United States as compared with what would be saved in health care costs after immunization? For example, it is estimated that for every dollar spent immunizing children with the measles-mumps-rubella vaccine, about 14 dollars are saved in health care costs. This is not the case for varicella, where one dollar spent on the vaccine saves about 90 cents in health care costs. However, if you consider that mothers and fathers miss work taking care of children with varicella, the dollar spent on varicella vaccine saves two dollars and 80 cents in cost to society. In part because of these societal costs, the varicella vaccine was recommended by the AAP two months after licensure by the FDA.

The issue of vaccine *use* is best shown by the hepatitis B vaccine (see Chapter 11 for more information). The hepatitis B vaccine was approved by the FDA in 1981. The decision by the ACIP at that time was to immunize groups only at high risk of acquiring hepatitis B virus infection, such as health care workers, intravenous drug users, homosexuals, and people living in the house of someone infected with hepatitis B. By 1991 it was clear that this strategy wasn't working: the number of cases and complications of hepatitis B virus infections in the United States remained unchanged. So the ACIP changed its strategy and has now recommended that all infants born in the United States receive the hepatitis B vaccine.

REQUIREMENT

The FDA, AAP, and ACIP do not *require* that vaccines be given to children.

Vaccines are required for school entry by state legislatures, and this requirement is enforced by state departments of health. Unlike the AAP and ACIP, states consider whether it is *practical* to require vaccines for all children within a state. This depends on whether there is enough of the vaccine available for all children within a particular age range, as well as whether there is enough vaccine provided at low cost by the federal government to allow immunization of children whose parents can't afford it.

For the most part, all vaccines that are recommended by the ACIP or AAP are required for school entry. However, there are state-to-state differences. For example, although the pertussis vaccine is recommended for use in all infants and young children by the ACIP and AAP, it is not required for school entry in Pennsylvania. The pertussis vaccine is, however, required for school entry in about 90 percent of states in the country. Parents should check with their local school districts to determine which vaccines are required for school entry.

THE RIGHT TO REFUSE VACCINES: PUBLIC HEALTH CONCERNS VS. INDIVIDUAL RIGHTS

In the United States there are exemptions to the vaccination requirement. For example, a subchapter of the Commonwealth of Pennsylvania's law requiring immunization for school entry reads as follows: "Children need not be immunized if the parent, guardian, or emancipated child objects in writing to the immunization on religious grounds or on the basis of a strong moral or ethical conviction similar to a religious belief."

The United States is different from many other countries in the recognition of the individual's right to refuse immunizations. There are, however, potential dangers in a country's decision to choose the rights of an individual above the rights of a group. Two examples are shown below:

- Between 1990 and 1991 in the city of Philadelphia, measles infected about 1,600 children and killed nine. Almost all of those cases and deaths occurred in children whose parents belonged to two churches that refused immunization based on religious grounds. The religious group refusing immunization was at the center of the measles epidemic and clearly was linked to the spread of measles to the surrounding community. Members of the religious group made a choice. They decided not to receive vaccines and, therefore, took the risk that their children might suffer severe and fatal infections. Their decision proved tragic not only for themselves, but also for other children in the community at risk of disease. Unfortunately, people in the surrounding community did not have a chance to participate in that decision.

- In 1978 and again in 1992, outbreaks of polio occurred in the Netherlands in members of a Dutch Reformed Church, a fundamentalist group that refused immunization for religious reasons. In the Netherlands the immunization rate against polio was about 97 percent. Not one case of polio occurred in people outside of the Dutch Reformed Church. However, not all countries have immunization rates this high. In the United States the immunization rate against polio is about 86 percent, and in some areas of this country it is as low as 35 percent. If an outbreak of polio were to occur in this country in a group that refused polio vaccine, it is not clear that we would be as lucky as the people in the Netherlands.

PART TWO

VACCINES FOR ALL CHILDREN

CHAPTER 6

WHEN DO CHILDREN GET VACCINES?

A Suggested Schedule for Vaccines			
Birth	*2 months*	*4 months*	*6 months*
Hepatitis B #1	DTaP #1	DTaP #2	DTaP #3
	Polio #1	Polio #2	Hib #3
	Hib #1	Hib #2	
	Hepatitis B #2		
12 months	*15 months*	*18 months*	*4 years*
MMR #1 (measles, mumps, rubella)	Hib #4	Polio #3	MMR #2
	Hepatitis B #3	DTaP #4	
Varicella			

5 years	*11–12 years*
DTaP #5	Td
Polio #4	

Vaccines are usually recommended to be given within a range of ages. For example, the first of three hepatitis B shots can be administered between birth and 2 months of age. In the suggested schedule above, we have chosen specific ages to give a number of vaccines. There are several advantages to this schedule:

- We recommend that the first hepatitis B vaccine be given at birth. Vaccinating at birth will help protect those children whose mothers are unknowingly infected with hepatitis B virus at the time of delivery (see Chapter 11 for more details).

- We recommend that the inactivated (or "killed") polio vaccine be given for the first two doses. This will significantly reduce the number of cases of paralysis caused by the vaccine (see Chapter 8 for more details).

- We recommend that the varicella vaccine be given at 12 months of age. By giving the varicella vaccine as soon as possible, the child is less likely to catch chickenpox before receiving the vaccine. Once the child catches natural (or "wild-type") chickenpox, it's too late. The "wild-type" virus will live silently in the child's nervous system and is more likely to cause severe shingles down the road than the vaccine virus (see Chapter 12 for more details).

- We recommend that the hepatitis B and Hib vaccines be given at 2 and 15 months of age because they can be combined as a single shot.

- We recommend that the MMR vaccine be given at the same time as the varicella vaccine. The MMR and varicella vaccines will soon be available as a single shot.

- We recommend that the DTaP and Hib vaccines be given at the same time, because a combined vaccine will soon be available for all doses.

These recommendations will change as different combination vaccines become available over the next several years (see Chapter 27).

DTaP (DIPHTHERIA-TETANUS-ACELLULAR PERTUSSIS)

Rachel is 2 months old. Her mother takes her to the doctor and finds out that there is a new vaccine. The vaccine that used to be called DTP is now called DTaP. This new vaccine, which prevents whooping cough (or pertussis) among other bacteria, is now supposedly purer and safer.

Is the new pertussis vaccine safe?

Was the old pertussis vaccine unsafe?

If there really is a question of safety, might it be best if Rachel didn't get any of the pertussis vaccines?

The letters *DTaP* stand for *D*iphtheria-*T*etanus-*a*cellular *P*ertussis. No vaccine has been more controversial than pertussis (whooping cough). This is because the old pertussis vaccine (included in the DTP vaccine) had a high rate of side effects. About 50 percent of children given this vaccine had low-grade fever or pain and soreness where the shot was given. The vaccine was also, albeit rarely, associated with severe side effects such as high fever, seizures, and persistent crying. Although the vaccine was remarkably effective in reducing the number of cases of pertussis, some parents were frightened enough that they hesitated to immunize their children.

Unfortunately, the biggest problem with the old pertussis vaccine was that it had bad press. Newspaper articles and television programs incorrectly linked it to diseases such as unexplained coma, sudden infant death syndrome (SIDS), epilepsy, and permanent brain damage. And some television programs claimed that there were "bad lots" of the DTP vaccine.

Fears of pertussis vaccine have been lessened by a new vaccine that includes a highly purified pertussis component called acellular pertussis. This vaccine was recommended for use in all children in 1997. In this chapter we will talk about the differences between the "old" DTP vaccine and the "new" DTaP vaccine and try to dispel some of the myths and fears that surround the pertussis vaccine.

Recommendation by the American Academy of Pediatrics

The American Academy of Pediatrics recommends that all children receive the DTaP vaccine as a series of five shots given at 2 months, 4 months, 6 months, 15 to 18 months, and 4 to 6 years of age.

PERTUSSIS

WHAT IS PERTUSSIS?

Pertussis, commonly called whooping cough, is a disease caused by a bacterium (*Bordetella pertussis*). Children with pertussis develop thick, sticky mucus in the windpipe, which causes severe spells of coughing often lasting two to three weeks. Sometimes the child coughs five to ten times before breathing in; when the child finally does breathe in there is often a loud gasp or "whooping" sound. Pertussis can also cause severe pneumonia and seizures.

Before the vaccine there were about 200,000 cases of pertussis, causing 8,000 deaths each year in the United States. Now there are about 6,000 reported cases of pertussis, causing only 10 deaths each year.

Pertussis Is One of the Most Contagious Diseases Known to Man

Ninety percent of unvaccinated children living with someone with pertussis will get sick. Fifty to 80 percent of unvaccinated children in school with someone with pertussis will get sick.

WHAT IS THE PERTUSSIS VACCINE?

Pertussis is caused by a protein (called a toxin) released by the bacteria as well as proteins that are part of the bacteria. Protection against pertussis depends in part upon making antibodies to the toxin as well as to these other bacterial proteins.

The "old" pertussis vaccine (called "whole-cell" vaccine) was made by taking the pertussis bacteria and growing them in broth (a nutrient-rich fluid in which bacteria grow). While growing in the broth, the bacteria would produce toxin. Then both the whole bacteria and the toxin were inactivated with formaldehyde. This whole-cell pertussis vaccine was used in the vaccine called DTP.

There is a big difference between the "new" pertussis vaccine (called acellular pertussis, or aP, vaccine) and the "old" DTP vaccine. The "new" vaccine is made by purifying both the toxin and individual bacterial proteins. The whole bacteria (or whole cell) is not present. That is why this pertussis vaccine is called "acellular." The purified toxin and bacterial proteins are then inactivated with a chemical, such as formaldehyde. The new, purer form of the pertussis vaccine is in the formulation called DTaP.

Are the DTP and DTaP vaccines safe?

Until recently, children were given the DTP vaccine. Now the DTaP vaccine is recommended.

The "old" DTP vaccine had a high rate of mild side effects (see Chapter 4). Most of the side effects were caused by the pertussis part of the vaccine. The DTP vaccine caused pain, swelling, and redness where the shot was given in up to 50 percent of children. In addition, the vaccine commonly caused low-grade fever, fretfulness, drowsiness, and vomiting. The DTaP vaccine was made to reduce this high rate of side effects. With this vaccine, the rate of these generally mild side effects has decreased from as high as 50 percent to between 1 and 5 percent.

The old DTP vaccine also had some side effects that were more worrisome. The DTP vaccine caused high fevers (0.3 percent), persistent crying (1 percent), and seizures (0.6 percent). These side effects were not permanent. With the new DTaP vaccine, their incidence is dramatically lower.

Unfortunately, the more unpleasant side effects of the "old" DTP vaccine discouraged some parents from giving pertussis vaccine to their children. The DTaP vaccine should relieve those concerns.

Did the "old" DTP vaccine cause epilepsy?

This question has probably received more attention from the media than all other vaccine-related topics. Although the answer is easy, understanding it is a little harder.

The "old" DTP vaccine clearly caused seizures. The risk was about one case per 1,750 doses. However, there is no evidence that the DTP vaccine caused epilepsy (a permanent seizure disorder). When children who had a seizure from the vaccine were compared ten years later with children who had not, there was no difference between groups in the incidence of epilepsy. Similarly, there was no difference in the incidence of epilepsy in children who had received the DTP vaccine as compared to those who had never received it. Therefore, although the DTP vaccine can trigger the first seizure in children who have epilepsy, the vaccine does not cause epilepsy.

The incidence of seizures with the "new" DTaP vaccine is dramatically lower than the "old" DTP vaccine. Several studies have found an incidence of seizures from the DTaP vaccine of 0 percent.

Did the "old" DTP vaccine cause seizures?

There is a problem that affects 2 to 4 percent of all children: febrile seizures. For whatever reasons, some children have seizures when they get fever. For these children, any illness that causes fever has the potential to cause seizures. In children with febrile seizures, the fever is usually from viral infections that cause colds, sore throats, vomiting, or diarrhea. The good news is that febrile seizures don't cause a permanent seizure disorder (epilepsy) and don't cause brain damage. Children usually grow out of having febrile seizures by 5 or 6 years of age.

Because vaccines can occasionally cause fever, they can also cause febrile seizures. The "old" DTP vaccine caused high fever (above 104.5°F) in about 0.3 percent of children. Therefore, it is not surprising that it was occasionally associated with febrile seizures. The incidence of fever with the "new" DTaP vaccine is about 5 to 10 times less than with the "old" DTP. Therefore, the incidence of febrile seizures associated with this vaccine will also be much lower.

Did the "old" DTP vaccine cause Sudden Infant Death Syndrome (SIDS)?

SIDS causes about 5,000 to 6,000 deaths each year in the United States. Because the disease affects children between 2 and 4 months of age, there is often a temporal relationship between the receipt of a DTP vaccine and SIDS. However, several studies performed over the past 10 years comparing children who received the DTP vaccine with those who did not receive it proved that the DTP vaccine did *not* cause SIDS.

Wasn't there a "bad lot" of the DTP vaccine?

Television news shows reported that there were "bad lots" of the DTP vaccine. Reports went as far as showing the lot number of the vaccine. Although these reports generated an understandable amount of anxiety among parents and physicians, there has never been any evidence that such "bad lots" actually existed.

The Food and Drug Administration (FDA) has the authority to withdraw lots of vaccines if there are questions about the vaccines' safety or effectiveness (potency). For example, in 1996–1997 the FDA withdrew several lots of the influenza vaccine because of reduced potency. The FDA has never recalled a lot of pertussis vaccine because of problems with the vaccine's safety.

Why can't I just avoid possible problems from the pertussis vaccine by not giving it?

Other countries have at times stopped giving the pertussis vaccine. For example, bad publicity about the vaccine in Japan caused people to stop using it there in 1975.

In the three years before the vaccine was stopped, there were 400 cases of pertussis, causing 10 deaths. In the three years after it was stopped, there were 13,000 cases of pertussis, causing 113 deaths. The frightening consequences of discontinuing the pertussis vaccine caused the Japanese to resume giving it in the early 1980s.

An Example of What Happens When You Stop Using the Pertussis Vaccine

	Cases of pertussis	Deaths from pertussis
Japan 1971–1974	400	10
Japan 1976–1979	13,000	113

My son was recently in the hospital with whooping cough. At the time our whole family was coughing. Can adults catch whooping cough too?

Pertussis has been shown to be a much more serious problem in adolescents and adults than was previously recognized. In fact, children usually catch pertussis from adult family members. Unfortunately, adolescents and adults injected with the "old" DTP vaccine had a high rate (about 80 to 90 percent) of soreness, tenderness, redness, and swelling at the site of injection. The "new" DTaP vaccine will probably lessen that problem, and there may soon be a time when adolescents and adults are routinely immunized against pertussis.

Pertussis Vaccine: Summary and Conclusions

The Chance of Catching Pertussis

There are about 6,000 cases of pertussis, causing ten deaths, reported to the Centers for Disease Control and Prevention each year in the United States.

The Risk of Serious Side Effects from the Pertussis Vaccine

The "old" pertussis vaccine (included in the vaccine called DTP) had a high rate of mild side effects. Most of the side effects were caused by the pertussis part of the vaccine. The DTP vaccine caused pain, swelling, and redness where the shot was given as well as fretfulness, drowsiness, vomiting, and low-grade fevers in up to 50 percent of children.

The "new" pertussis vaccine (included in the vaccine called DTaP) is much purer and was made to reduce this high rate of side effects. With the "new" DTaP vaccine, the rate of these generally mild side effects has decreased dramatically from about 50 percent to between 1 and 5 percent.

In addition, the DTP vaccine occasionally caused severe side effects, including persistent crying (in 1 percent of cases), seizures (0.6 percent), and high fever (0.3 percent). None of these side effects were permanent. With the DTaP vaccine, the incidence of these side effects is dramatically lower.

Conclusions

The "old" pertussis vaccine was rarely a cause of severe side effects, including seizures. The "new," purer pertussis vaccine has significantly reduced and in some instances eliminated these rare side effects.

In any case, the benefits of receiving even the "old" pertussis vaccine clearly outweighed the risks of not taking it. Because of the negative publicity surrounding the pertussis vaccine, its use was essentially discontinued in both England and Japan in the mid-1970s and early 1980s.

Many children died of severe pertussis infection as a direct result of stopping the vaccine. On the other hand, no child has died from the "old" pertussis vaccine.

The use of a "new" pertussis vaccine will only enhance the benefit-to-risk ratio.

DIPHTHERIA

WHAT IS DIPHTHERIA?

Diphtheria is caused by a toxin that is released by a bacterium (*Corynebacterium diphtheriae*). The toxin causes a thick, gray coating at the back of the throat that makes it difficult for a child to breathe or swallow. The bacterium also produces a harmful protein (called toxin) that can invade the heart, kidneys, and nerves. About one out of every ten children with diphtheria infection will die from suffocation, heart failure, or paralysis.

Before the vaccine there were as many as 200,000 cases of diphtheria, causing 15,000 deaths each year in the United States. Because of the vaccine, there are now only about two cases of diphtheria each year. Between 1980 and 1995, only four children died from diphtheria.

WHAT IS THE DIPHTHERIA VACCINE?

Diphtheria causes disease by making a toxin that is released by the bacteria. Protection against diphtheria depends upon manufacturing antibodies to this toxin.

The diphtheria vaccine is made by taking the toxin, purifying it, and inactivating it with the chemical formaldehyde. An inactivated toxin is called a toxoid. Toxoids cause immunity without causing disease.

Why should I give my child a vaccine for a disease I've never even heard of?

There was a time when diphtheria was a devastating and feared illness. In 1920 there were 148,000 cases of diphtheria in the United States. In Canada, it was the leading cause of death in school-aged children.

Because of the vaccine, the incidence of diphtheria has decreased from a peak of 148,000 cases to two cases a year. However, we should not be made complacent by this remarkable success. For example, each year there are outbreaks of diphtheria in eastern Europe, Russia, Brazil, Nigeria, India, Indonesia, and the Philippines. The outbreaks of diphtheria that occurred in eastern Europe and Russia were due to a severe decrease in immunization rates among children in those countries. If we stop giving the vaccine in this country, the disease will be heard from again.

DIPHTHERIA VACCINE: SUMMARY AND CONCLUSIONS

THE CHANCE OF CATCHING DIPHTHERIA

Diphtheria is an extremely rare cause of disease in the United States. Only about three to five cases are reported each year. Between 1980 and 1995, four children in the United States died from diphtheria.

THE RISK OF SERIOUS SIDE EFFECTS FROM THE DIPHTHERIA VACCINE

There are no serious side effects from the diphtheria vaccine.

CONCLUSIONS

Over the past 16 years, there have been 41 cases of diphtheria and four deaths; no child has died from the diphtheria vaccine. Therefore, the risk of severe disease caused by diptheria is extremely small, and the risk of serious side effects from the diphtheria vaccine is probably zero.

In addition, when you consider that major outbreaks of severe and fatal diphtheria infections continue to occur in eastern Europe and Russia, and that these outbreaks were due to a decrease in immunization rates among children, it clearly pays to maintain an immunized population of children against this rare but deadly infection.

TETANUS

WHAT IS TETANUS?

Tetanus is also a disease caused by a bacterium (*Clostridium tetani*). The tetanus bacteria live in the soil and may enter the skin through a cut or puncture wound. Once under the skin, the bacteria can make a toxin that causes severe and painful spasms of the muscles.

Sometimes tetanus can be fatal. Muscle spasms of the throat can block the windpipe and cause instant death from suffocation. Also, the tetanus toxin can cause severe damage to the heart.

Before the vaccine there were about 600 cases of tetanus causing 180 deaths each year in the United States. Now there are about 70 cases of tetanus causing 15 deaths each year.

A Vaccine for a Disease That Isn't Contagious

The tetanus vaccine is unusual. Tetanus is one of the few vaccines given to prevent a disease that is not contagious. The deadly tetanus bacteria come from the soil and not from another person.

WHAT IS THE TETANUS VACCINE?

Like diphtheria, tetanus causes disease by making a toxin that is released by the bacteria. Protection against tetanus depends upon producing antibodies to this toxin.

The tetanus vaccine is made by taking the toxin, purifying it, and inactivating it with the chemical formaldehyde.

Can't I avoid tetanus by simply washing cuts very carefully?

Although careful washing of cuts and puncture wounds is important, this does not ensure protection against tetanus. Sometimes it is not possible to reach bacteria under the skin after a deep puncture wound.

Does the series of five DTaP shots protect my children against these diseases for the rest of their lives?

No. Protection from these vaccines often decreases over several years. Therefore, the diphtheria and tetanus vaccines should be given about every ten years for the rest of your life. These vaccines (in a preparation called Td) are recommended to be given starting at 11 to 12 years of age. This is the recommended age for adolescents to visit the doctor for vaccines (see Chapter 32 for details).

Vaccines Aren't Just for Kids

The diphtheria and tetanus vaccine (called Td) should be given every ten years beginning at about 11 to 12 years of age.

My 14-year-old daughter recently cut herself on a piece of glass while walking barefoot in our backyard. Should she get the tetanus vaccine?

A tetanus vaccine should be given to a child who has a cut likely to be contaminated with tetanus bacteria (for example, puncture wounds contaminated with dirt, soil, or saliva). These children do not need a tetanus vaccine if they have received at least three doses of tetanus vaccine *and* have been immunized within the past five years.

TETANUS VACCINE: SUMMARY AND CONCLUSIONS

THE CHANCE OF CATCHING TETANUS

Every year in the United States, 70 cases of tetanus causing 15 deaths are reported to the Centers for Disease Control and Prevention. Most of these cases occur in elderly adults.

THE RISK OF SERIOUS SIDE EFFECTS FROM THE TETANUS VACCINE

There are no serious side effects from the tetanus vaccine.

CONCLUSIONS

There are no risks from the tetanus vaccine, but there *is* a very real risk of severe and fatal tetanus infection. Therefore, all children should receive the tetanus vaccine. In addition, because the disease occurs most commonly in the elderly, it is important to get the tetanus vaccine (given with the diphtheria vaccine in a preparation called Td) every ten years starting at about 11 to 12 years of age.

CHAPTER 8

POLIO

Andy is 2 months old. His mother takes him to the doctor and finds out that there are two different polio vaccines. One vaccine is given as drops in the mouth and the other is a shot.

The doctor says there is now a change in the way that the polio vaccines are given. He says that the change was made because on very rare occasions children were paralyzed by the vaccine that was given as drops. Children are now supposed to get the polio shot at 2 and 4 months of age followed by the polio drops at about 15 months and 4 years of age. The doctor says that alternatively Andy could get all four doses as shots or all four doses as drops.

The doctor tells Andy's mother that the decision of whether to give the shot or the drops is hers. What should she do?

There are two different polio virus vaccines. One is a live, weakened virus that is given as drops in the mouth (the oral polio vaccine, or OPV). The other is a killed virus that is given as a shot (the inactivated polio vaccine, or IPV). For 35 years, virtually all children have been given only OPV. Recently that recommendation changed.

In October of 1996, the Centers for Disease Control and Prevention (CDC) recommended that instead of receiving four successive doses of

OPV, all children should now receive two doses of IPV followed by two doses of OPV.

Many parents are now confused by the choice between these two polio vaccines. In this chapter we will talk about why there are two vaccines and which one we think is best.

Recommendation by the Centers for Disease Control and Prevention (CDC)

The CDC recommends that all children receive the inactivated polio vaccine (IPV) as a shot given at 2 and 4 months of age, followed by the oral polio vaccine (OPV) given as drops in the mouth at 12 to 18 months and 4 to 6 years of age. However, using the same schedule of dosing, either four doses of OPV or four doses of IPV are considered acceptable alternatives.

What Is Polio?

Polio is caused by a virus. Most people who become infected with natural (or "wild-type") polio virus never get sick. Others will have a sore throat, cough, fever, stomach pain, vomiting, or a stiff neck and headache.

About one out of every thousand people who get natural polio infection will be paralyzed. Usually the legs and arms are paralyzed, but the muscles that assist breathing can become paralyzed too.

Before the polio vaccine, there were 13,000 to 20,000 people paralyzed and about 1,000 people killed each year in the United States by polio. Most of these victims were elementary school children.

Because of polio vaccine (first given in the United States in 1954), natural polio virus infections have been eliminated from this country.

The Horror of Polio

"During her first night in the hospital, when the virus had raged through her body, deadening muscle after muscle but leaving

continues

her body on fire with pain, doctors had performed an emergency tracheotomy to keep her from suffocating. . . .

"Her throat muscles useless, she was unable to breathe, cough or swallow on her own. . . . Mother was among the sickest, highest-risk polio patients."

From Kathryn Black's *In the Shadow of Polio*, 1996

WHAT IS THE POLIO VACCINE?

There are two polio virus vaccines: the oral polio vaccine (OPV) (given as a pink liquid by mouth) and the inactivated polio vaccine (IPV) (given as a shot). To know how these two polio vaccines work, you need to know how the polio virus makes children sick.

The polio virus first infects a child after entering the mouth and then grows, or replicates, in the intestines. The virus then leaves the intestines, enters the bloodstream, and sometimes travels to the brain and spinal cord (the nervous system). Once in the nervous system, the virus replicates again, damages the nerves, and causes paralysis. Polio grows in the intestines or in the nervous system according to an internal blueprint (the genes).

OPV is made by changing the blueprint so that the virus can still grow in the intestines but can't grow in the nervous system. Because OPV is given by mouth, antibodies are made at the intestinal surface as well as in the blood. Because the intestines are the first place the polio virus grows, OPV creates a first line of defense in the intestines against future polio infections.

IPV is made by killing the virus with the chemical formaldehyde. IPV is given as a shot and causes antibodies to be made in the bloodstream, but less so in the intestines. Because natural polio goes into the bloodstream only after it has replicated in the intestines, IPV creates a second line of defense in the bloodstream against future polio infections.

OPV and IPV Work Differently

Here's another way to think about the differences between these two vaccines.

continues

Let's say one child got OPV and another child was given IPV. Both children come in contact with a third child, who is infected with natural polio and is highly contagious.

The child given OPV has antibodies present at his intestinal surface and in his blood. When he is exposed to polio, his intestinal antibodies will not let polio grow in his intestines. Therefore, the child given OPV will not be paralyzed by polio. In addition, polio virus will not grow in his intestines, possibly spreading the disease to someone else.

On the other hand, the child who was given IPV primarily has antibodies in her bloodstream. Because of this, she will also not be paralyzed by polio. But because she doesn't have as many antibodies in her intestines as children receiving OPV, polio may still grow in her intestines and spread to another child.

So both vaccines can prevent paralysis from polio, but OPV is better than IPV at stopping the spread of polio among children.

Why are there two polio vaccines?

The first polio vaccine made in this country was IPV. This vaccine, made by Dr. Jonas Salk, was first given in 1954. Because of the Salk vaccine, the number of cases of paralysis from polio decreased from 20,000 in 1952 to 2,500 in 1960.

The second polio vaccine made was OPV. This vaccine was made by Dr. Albert Sabin and was first given in the United States in 1961.

By 1963 there were two polio vaccines available in the United States. As a result, this country was faced with a decision. Which of these two vaccines should we use?

OPV was chosen for four reasons:

1. OPV worked better than IPV at that time. One hundred percent of children given OPV were protected against natural polio, as compared to about 90 percent given the IPV.

2. OPV was better than IPV at stopping the spread of polio (see the box above).

3. OPV caused immunity lasting longer than that of IPV.

4. Children immunized with OPV often spread the vaccine virus (and consequently immunity) to other children and adults living in the home (known as "herd immunity").

As it turned out, the decision in 1963 to recommend only OPV was the right one. Epidemics of polio were stopped, and there has not been a case of paralysis from natural polio virus in the United States since 1979.

Are the polio vaccines safe?

IPV is completely safe. A small number of children given this vaccine may have pain where the shot was given.

OPV, on the other hand, has an extremely rare but very dangerous side effect. About one in 750,000 children given their first dose of OPV will either become paralyzed or spread the altered vaccine virus to someone living in the home or community who will become paralyzed.

Every year in the United States, the oral polio vaccine causes about eight to ten cases of permanent paralysis.

How Does OPV Cause Paralysis?

OPV is made by the process of cell-culture adaptation. The way this is done is as follows:

Polio virus normally grows in cells that line the human intestine or in cells that make up the human nervous system. In order to alter the virus so that it can no longer grow in the nervous system, polio virus is adapted to growth in specialized cells grown in the laboratory. This adaptation causes a series of genetic mutations that no longer allow the virus to grow in the nervous system.

However, OPV still grows very well in the human intestine. Very rarely, when OPV is growing in the intestines, a series of genetic mutations occur that involves those same genes that determine nervous system growth. When that happens, the vaccine virus is said to have reverted to "wild-type" virus and is again capable of causing paralysis.

Why did the polio vaccine recommendation change?

In the early 1950s there were epidemics of polio every year. In 1955, IPV was introduced in the United States and the incidence of paralysis from polio was reduced by 90 percent; epidemics were virtually halted by the end of the decade. OPV became available in 1961, and, since then, has been the nation's primary polio vaccine.

However, two important things have happened since the 1950s that have led to the change in the polio vaccine recommendation. First, the polio virus has not only been eliminated from this country, it has been eliminated from the Western Hemisphere—there has not been a case of polio in the United States since 1979 or in the Americas since 1991. Second, IPV has been improved.

The new IPV is called *eIPV*, which stands for *e*nhanced-potency *i*nactivated *p*olio *v*accine. The new inactivated vaccine is enhanced in that there is a greater quantity of purified, killed polio virus in the preparation. The greater quantity of virus induces both greater quantities of virus-specific antibodies and a higher level of protection against polio disease than was seen with the original Salk vaccine.

Which of the polio vaccines should I give my children?

We agree that the recommendation to give the sequence of two doses of IPV followed by two doses of OPV is the best choice. Almost all of the paralysis from OPV happens after the first two doses. By using IPV for the first and second doses, this rare problem will be largely eliminated. Also by giving OPV for the third and fourth doses, infants will still benefit from the long-lasting immunity and the "first line of defense" that OPV provides.

We also agree that using four successive doses of IPV alone would be an acceptable choice. A number of countries including France, The Netherlands, Canada, Finland, Norway, and Sweden use only IPV. France is probably most similar to the United States in that both countries admit many tourists and immigrants from countries where natural polio infections still exist. France appears to have successfully eliminated natural polio by using only IPV; there has not been a case of polio there since 1989.

The new recommendation still includes the use of live polio virus. Doesn't that mean that my child could still be paralyzed?

One hundred percent of children given the first dose of OPV will shed OPV in their feces (often for several weeks). The second time children get OPV, only about 40 percent will shed OPV, and after the third dose only about 10 percent will shed it. Because IPV is inactivated, no children shed polio virus after receiving IPV.

The question is whether the new IPV decreases the percentage of children who shed OPV after getting OPV. The surprising answer is yes. Only about 20 percent of children given two doses of the new IPV will shed OPV after receiving OPV for the first time.

Therefore, receiving IPV significantly decreases the chance that OPV will successfully grow in the intestines and revert to natural polio virus.

If we don't see polio anymore in this country, why should I give my child any of the polio vaccines?

Although the polio virus has been eliminated from the Western Hemisphere, it has not been eliminated from the rest of the world. Outbreaks of polio continue to occur in Asia and Africa. Because global travel is more widespread now than ever, an outbreak of polio in this country could be imported.

The World Health Organization, through extensive worldwide use of OPV, has targeted polio virus for elimination by the year 2003. If that goal is achieved, polio vaccines, like the smallpox vaccine, will eventually be considered unnecessary.

POLIO VACCINE:
SUMMARY AND CONCLUSIONS
THE CHANCE OF CATCHING POLIO

There has not been a case of natural or "wild-type" polio in the United States since 1979 or in the Western Hemisphere since 1991. The only real chance of catching polio is through contact with an infected person who travels to this country.

Therefore, the chance of catching polio in this country approaches zero.

THE RISK OF SERIOUS SIDE EFFECTS FROM THE POLIO VACCINE

The oral polio vaccine, or OPV, causes eight to ten cases of paralysis every year in the United States either in recipients of the vaccine or in contacts of children who have received it (almost all of these cases are associated with receipt of the first two doses of OPV).

The inactivated polio vaccine, or IPV, does not have serious side effects.

CONCLUSIONS

In the United States the risk of paralysis from the oral polio vaccine is greater than the risk of paralysis from natural polio. Therefore, the Centers for Disease Control and Prevention have recently recommended that the first two doses of polio vaccine should be with IPV and the next two doses with OPV. If IPV is given first, the incidence of paralysis following OPV will likely be curtailed or eliminated.

We also fully support the use of a four-dose IPV schedule. We recommend an all-OPV schedule for those infants likely to live or travel for months in southeast Asia or Africa.

Chapter 9

HIB ("THE MENINGITIS VACCINE")

Jessica is 2 months old. Her mother is told by the doctor that she will be getting a vaccine called "Hib" that prevents meningitis. Does this mean that Jessica will never catch meningitis?

Hib stands for *Haemophilus influenzae* type b, a bacterium that is a common cause of bacterial meningitis. This vaccine was licensed for use in all children less than 5 years old in 1990, and the results have been dramatic. Cases of Hib meningitis in the United States have decreased from 13,000 per year to fewer than 100, and deaths from Hib meningitis have decreased from 500 a year to fewer than five.

Recommendation by the American Academy of Pediatrics

The Hib vaccine is recommended to be given as a series of shots to all children under 5 years of age.

There are three pharmaceutical companies that make the Hib vaccine used for infants. Two of the vaccines are given as a series of four shots at 2, 4, 6, and 12 to 15 months of age. One Hib vaccine is given as a series of three shots at 2, 4, and 12 to 15 months of age.

WHAT IS HIB?

Haemophilus influenzae type b (Hib) infects the lining of the brain, causing meningitis. The infection begins with high fever, decreased appetite, and irritability. The child then becomes drowsy and may get a stiff neck or a headache. Hib can also cause sepsis (bloodstream infection), with symptoms of fever, low blood pressure, and shock. Usually Hib infects children under 2 years of age.

Even though we have antibiotics to treat Hib, one out of every 20 children with Hib meningitis will die from the disease. Also, about one out of every five children who survive Hib meningitis will be left blind, deaf, mentally retarded, or learning disabled. Obviously, it makes more sense to prevent Hib meningitis with a vaccine than to treat it with an antibiotic.

Hib can also cause severe swelling of a tissue (the epiglottis) that helps close the windpipe when we swallow. Children with infection of the epiglottis (called epiglottitis) can die from suffocation. In addition, Hib can cause severe infection of the joints (arthritis) and bones (osteomyelitis).

Is Meningitis Contagious?

Yes! Young children exposed to a brother or sister with Hib infection are 500 times more likely to get meningitis than children whose siblings are not infected.

WHAT IS THE HIB VACCINE?

The Hib bacterium is coated with a sugar called polysaccharide. To be protected against Hib, you need immunity to this sugar. Unfortunately, infants and children under 2 years of age can't develop immunity to this sugar. Even children who get Hib meningitis at a young age are not immune after infection. However, researchers found that if you join the sugar to a harmless protein (in a conjugate vaccine), children develop immunity to the sugar and are protected against Hib.

Before the Hib vaccine, there were about 13,000 cases of Hib meningitis, causing 400 to 500 deaths each year in the United States. Hib meningitis was the leading cause of acquired mental retardation in the United States.

The current Hib vaccines in this country were first licensed in 1990, and the incidence of Hib infections has been dramatically reduced. As a measure of the importance of the Hib vaccine, four scientists associated with its development were awarded the 1996 Nobel Prize for Medicine.

Before and After the Hib Vaccine		
	Before the vaccine (1980)	*After the vaccine (1995)*
Infections	25,000	1,300
Meningitis	13,000	86
Deaths	400–500	5

Is the Hib vaccine safe?

Yes. The only symptoms are mild. After receiving the Hib vaccine, about 10 to 15 percent of children will develop pain or soreness where the shot was given, and about 2 percent of children will have low-grade fever.

The Hib Vaccine Is Unique

Immunity after Hib vaccination is better than immunity after Hib infection. Only the Hib and tetanus vaccines can make that claim.

Will the Hib vaccine prevent my child from getting meningitis?

Meningitis is also caused by other viruses and bacteria. However, meningitis is much more likely to be deadly or cause permanent brain damage if it is caused by a bacterium than if it is caused by a virus.

Before the vaccine, Hib was the most common cause of bacterial meningitis in children. So the Hib vaccine doesn't prevent all cases of meningitis, but it does prevent the formerly most common cause of severe meningitis.

Since the Hib vaccine became available, the two most common causes of bacterial meningitis are pneumococcus and meningococcus. For a description of the vaccines against these infections, see Part 3, "Vaccines for Some Children."

Will the Hib vaccine prevent my child from getting ear infections or sinusitis?

No. Hib is not a likely cause of either ear infections or sinusitis.

HIB VACCINE:
SUMMARY AND CONCLUSIONS

THE CHANCE OF CATCHING HIB

Because of the Hib vaccine, the chances of catching the Hib bacterium, which causes inflammation of the lining of the brain (meningitis), bloodstream infection (sepsis), and pneumonia, have been dramatically reduced.

THE RISK OF SERIOUS SIDE EFFECTS FROM THE HIB VACCINE

There are no serious side effects from the Hib vaccine.

CONCLUSIONS

There are no risks of serious side effects from the Hib vaccine, but there is a small risk of getting a Hib infection. Because infection with Hib is often severe and occasionally fatal, all children should receive the Hib vaccine.

CHAPTER 10

MMR (MEASLES-MUMPS-RUBELLA)

Joseph is 15 years old. Joseph's mother recently discovered that there is an outbreak of measles in his high school.

Joseph got a measles vaccine when he was 1 year old. Will the vaccine Joseph received 14 years ago protect him from getting measles at school?

Why are all children these days getting two doses of the measles vaccine instead of one?

The letters *MMR* stand for *M*easles-*M*umps-*R*ubella.

The combination of measles, mumps, and rubella ("German measles") vaccines has been around for about 25 years and has had an amazing impact on the health of children.

Because of the MMR vaccine, the incidence of deaths in the United States caused by measles has decreased from 3,000 a year to almost none, of encephalitis (inflammation of the brain) caused by mumps virus from 400 a year to fewer than five, and of birth defects and mental retardation caused by rubella from 20,000 a year to two.

63

Recommendation by the American Academy of Pediatrics

The MMR vaccine is recommended to be given in the form of two shots. The first shot is given at 12 to 15 months of age, and the second shot is given at 4 to 6 years of age.

MEASLES

WHAT IS MEASLES?

Measles is a disease caused by a virus. It usually begins with a cough, runny nose, fever, and "pink eye." A rash then appears on the face, spreads to the rest of the body, and lasts for about five days. Many children develop severe water loss (or dehydration) from the infection.

A devastating consequence of measles is pneumonia, affecting about 5 percent of young children infected with the virus. In Philadelphia, nine children died of measles between 1990 and 1991; most of them died of pneumonia. None of these children had received the measles vaccine.

In older children, measles can cause an infection of the brain called encephalitis, which can lead to brain damage. Although only about one out of every thousand children infected with measles develops encephalitis, 25 percent of those children will have permanent brain damage.

Before the vaccine, there were about 3 to 4 million cases of measles, causing 3,000 deaths, each year in the United States. Now there are about 300 to 500 cases of measles each year and almost no reported deaths.

WHAT IS THE MEASLES VACCINE?

The measles virus normally grows in cells that line the back of a child's throat and in cells lining the lungs. The measles vaccine was made by taking measles virus from the throat of an infected child and adapting it to grow in specialized cells grown in the laboratory. The cells in which measles virus vaccine was grown were chick embryo cells. As the virus became better and better able to grow in chick embryo cells, it became less and less able to grow in a child's skin or lungs. When this cell-culture adapted virus (or vaccine virus) was given to children, it replicated only a little before it was eliminated from the body.

Because the measles virus can still replicate a little in the child (meaning the vaccine virus is still alive), it is called a live, weakened (or attenuated) vaccine.

Before and After the Measles Vaccine

	Before the vaccine (1962)	After the vaccine (1995)
Cases of measles	4,000,000	309
Hospitalizations	48,000	33
Deaths	3,000	0

Is the measles vaccine safe?

More than 240 million doses of measles vaccine were administered in the United States between 1963 and 1993. The record of safety for this vaccine is excellent.

Fever in excess of 103°F occurs in about 5 to 15 percent of immunized children. The fever usually begins five to twelve days after administration of the vaccine.

Rash develops in about 5 to 10 percent of immunized children and is short-lived. Some parents worry that this rash may mean that their child is contagious. However, the weakened measles virus (vaccine virus) is not detected in the throat, respiratory tract, or skin, and so far transmission of measles vaccine virus from one person to another has not been documented.

Because the measles virus is grown in chick embryo cells, children with egg allergies were at one time advised not to receive the vaccine. However, recent studies found that the measles vaccine *can* be given to children with severe egg allergies without serious side effects.

Hypersensitivity reactions (or anaphylaxis) are extremely rare after receipt of the combination MMR vaccine. Anaphylaxis consists of swelling of the mouth, difficulty breathing, low blood pressure, and, rarely, shock. Since reporting of all serious side effects from vaccines was implemented in the United States in 1990 (see Chapter 4), more than 70 million doses of the MMR vaccine have been distributed. Eleven cases of anaphylaxis (and no deaths) occurred immediately after administration of the MMR vaccine.

Measles in Colonial America

"That fatal and never to be forgotten year, 1759, when the Lord sent the destroying Angel to pass through this place, and removed many of our friends into eternity in a short space of time; and not a house exempt, not a family spared from the calamity. So dreadful was it, that it made every ear tingle, and every heart bleed; in which time I and my family were exercised with that dreadful disorder, the measles. But blessed by God our lives are spared."

From the diary of Ephraim Harris
of Fairfield, New Jersey, 1759.

Why do children now have to get two shots of the measles vaccine when they only used to get only one?

In 1989, the recommendation from the American Academy of Pediatrics changed from a single dose of measles vaccine at 12 to 15 months of age to two doses of the vaccine. The second dose is now given at 4 to 6 years of age. Ninety-five percent of children are immune after the first dose.

If the measles vaccine induces immunity in 95 percent of people after one dose, why give another? There were three reasons this change was made. First, only about 87 to 90 percent of children actually receive the measles vaccine. Therefore, a recommendation for a second dose provides many children with a second chance to receive their first dose of the vaccine. Second, about 5 percent of children who receive the first vaccine won't develop immunity; most of these children do develop immunity after the second dose. Third, children who had an immune response to the first dose of vaccine could get a "booster" effect (a further increase in antibodies) by getting a second dose.

The change in recommendation was to try to lower the number of children, adolescents, and young adults who still get measles.

Measles Virus Also Causes a Rare Disease Called SSPE

Subacute sclerosing panencephalitis, or SSPE, is a rare disease of the brain caused by measles virus. The disease begins about seven years after measles infection, when the child develops personality changes, seizures, weakness, brain damage, and coma, leading to death.

Before the measles vaccine, there were about 20 cases of SSPE every year. The measles vaccine has virtually eliminated this disease.

My son was recently accepted to college and told that he had to get the MMR vaccine. Does he really need it?

Measles outbreaks continue to occur in high schools and on college campuses. To make sure that young adults are protected at the time that they enter college, the Centers for Disease Control and Prevention have now instructed all states to require proof of either two doses of measles vaccine or evidence for past measles virus infection at the time of college entry.

MEASLES VACCINE: SUMMARY AND CONCLUSIONS

THE CHANCE OF CATCHING MEASLES

Measles outbreaks continue to occur in the United States every year. As recently as 1990, there were about 28,000 cases of measles and about 30 deaths. Virtually all of these cases occurred in unimmunized people.

As an extreme example, in 1990 to 1991, nine unimmunized children in Philadelphia died of measles virus pneumonia.

THE RISK OF SERIOUS SIDE EFFECTS FROM THE MEASLES VACCINE

The serious side effect of the measles vaccine is hypersensitivity (or anaphylaxis). Since 1990, when a system for reporting serious side effects from vaccines was established, there have been 11 cases of anaphylaxis (swelling of the mouth, hives, low blood pressure, or shock) associated with the 70 million doses of the measles vaccine. So far no one has died of anaphylaxis from the vaccine.

CONCLUSIONS

The chance of having serious or fatal measles disease is extremely low, but the chance of serious side effects or death from the measles vaccine is about zero. Therefore, the immediate benefit of the measles vaccine outweighs the risk. In addition, because measles virus still circulates in the United States, decreased use of the measles vaccine would likely result in a resurgence of measles in this country.

MUMPS

WHAT IS MUMPS?

Like measles, mumps is a disease caused by a virus. Mumps usually infects children younger than 10 years old and begins with swelling of the salivary glands, or parotid glands, that are just below the ear. The swelling usually lasts for about one week.

Mumps also causes an infection of the lining of the brain (meningitis) in about 50 percent of cases. Before the mumps vaccine, mumps virus was the most common cause of viral meningitis. Because infection of the brain was fairly common, mumps was also the most common cause of acquired deafness.

Up to 40 percent of males infected with mumps after the age of puberty develop a painful swelling of the testicles called orchitis. In rare cases, orchitis can lead to both sterility and testicular cancer.

In addition, there was an increase in fetal deaths in women who were infected with mumps virus in the first trimester of pregnancy.

Before the vaccine, there were about 200,000 cases of mumps, causing 20 to 30 deaths, each year in the United States. Now there are about 900 cases of mumps and no associated deaths each year.

WHAT IS THE MUMPS VACCINE?

The development of the mumps vaccine is described in detail in Chapter 3.

The mumps vaccine is made in a manner similar to that used to develop the measles vaccine. The mumps virus, which normally grows in cells of the salivary glands or cells that line the back of the throat, is instead grown in chick embryo cells. The virus is weakened when it grows in chicken cells so that it can no longer cause disease in children but can still create immunity.

Like the measles vaccine, the mumps vaccine is a live, weakened (or attenuated) virus.

Is the mumps vaccine safe?

The mumps vaccine is remarkably safe and is only a rare cause of low-grade fever or pain where the shot was given. Like the measles vaccine, it can be administered safely to children who are allergic to eggs.

MUMPS VACCINE: SUMMARY AND CONCLUSIONS

THE CHANCE OF CATCHING MUMPS

Each year in the United States there are about 900 cases of mumps and no associated deaths; probably half of the children infected with mumps will develop a mild infection of the lining of the brain (meningitis) or of the brain itself (encephalitis).

THE RISK OF SERIOUS SIDE EFFECTS FROM THE MUMPS VACCINE

The mumps vaccine is not associated with any serious side effects.

CONCLUSIONS

The chance of developing a serious mumps infection is extremely low, and the chance of having a serious reaction from the mumps vaccine is about zero. So the immediate benefit of mumps vaccine outweighs the risk. Also, because the mumps virus still circulates in the United States, decreased use of the vaccine would likely result in a resurgence of the disease.

RUBELLA

WHAT IS RUBELLA?

Rubella, better known as German measles, also is a disease caused by a virus. Rubella begins with fever, swollen glands, and a light rash on the face that looks like a mild case of measles. Although usually harmless, the rubella virus occasionally infects the brain, resulting in encephalitis, and causes a decrease in platelets, cells that help the blood to clot.

However, if a woman is infected with rubella virus during pregnancy the results are disastrous. Up to 85 percent of infants whose mothers are infected with rubella in the first three months of gestation will have blindness, deafness, heart defects, or mental retardation.

Between 1964 and 1965 there were about 12 million cases of rubella in the United States, causing birth defects in 20,000 children. Now that we have a vaccine, the number of children with birth defects caused by rubella virus has decreased to two cases per year.

> **Girls Are Immunized with Rubella Vaccine to Protect Their Future Children**
>
> Rubella vaccine is an example of vaccinating one person to protect another.
>
> *continues*

> We vaccinate girls so that if they become pregnant as adults, their unborn babies will be protected against the harmful effects of rubella virus.
> We vaccinate boys to help stop the spread of the virus.

WHAT IS THE RUBELLA VACCINE?

The rubella vaccine is made in a manner similar to both the measles and mumps vaccines. Rubella virus, which normally grows in cells that line the back of the throat, is grown instead in human fibroblast cells (fibroblasts help hold various tissues of the body together). The virus is weakened when it grows in these fibroblast cells so that it can no longer cause disease in children but can still cause immunity.

Like the measles and mumps vaccines, the rubella vaccine is a live, weakened (or attenuated) virus.

The Link Between Rubella Virus and Birth Defects

McAlistar Gregg was the first person to realize that rubella virus caused birth defects.

"In the first half of the year, 1941, an unusual number of cases of congenital cataracts made their appearance in Sydney. . . . By a calculation from the date of birth of the baby it was estimated that the early period of pregnancy corresponded with the . . . very widespread and severe epidemic in 1940 of the so-called German measles.

"In each new case it was found that the mother had suffered from that disease early in her pregnancy. . . . In some cases she had not at that time yet realized that she was pregnant."

From N. McAlister Gregg, an Australian ophthalmologist, 1941.

Is the rubella vaccine safe?

Low-grade fever occurs in about 1 percent of those vaccinated and a mild rash in about 5 percent. Children who have a rash from the rubella vaccine are not contagious and do not need to be isolated from pregnant women.

About 15 percent of adult women who are immunized with rubella vaccine will develop swelling and pain in the joints (arthritis). The arthritis is short-lived, or acute, and usually affects knees and fingers. This is not surprising when you consider that about 70 percent of adult women naturally infected with rubella will develop acute arthritis.

Fortunately, arthritis from the rubella vaccine is extremely rare in children younger than 14 years of age.

If a woman accidentally gets the rubella vaccine when she is pregnant, can her baby get birth defects?

So far there has never been a child who suffered birth defects because a rubella vaccine was given during pregnancy—and the vaccine has been mistakenly given during over 1,000 pregnancies. However, because it is theoretically possible that the rubella vaccine could cause birth defects, it should not be given to pregnant women.

Women who plan to conceive usually have their blood checked for the presence of antibodies to rubella as part of routine care. If a woman is not immune to rubella, she should receive the rubella vaccine at least three months prior to conception.

RUBELLA VACCINE: SUMMARY AND CONCLUSIONS

THE CHANCE OF CATCHING RUBELLA

Every year there are about 200 cases of rubella and two to three reported cases of birth defects caused by rubella infection during pregnancy.

THE RISK OF SERIOUS SIDE EFFECTS FROM THE RUBELLA VACCINE

The most serious side effect from rubella vaccine is the development of short-lived—less than one week, and not chronic—arthritis (or swelling of the joints). This occurs in as many as 15 percent of adult women who receive the vaccine. Fortunately, this complication occurs extremely rarely (probably less than 1 percent of the time) in children younger than 14 years of age who are given the rubella vaccine.

CONCLUSIONS

Since the introduction of the rubella vaccine, the incidence of birth defects caused by rubella infection during pregnancy has been extremely rare. About two to three children every year in the United States have blindness, deafness, heart defects, or mental retardation as a consequence of maternal rubella infection.

The serious side effect from the rubella vaccine is short-lived swelling of the joints.

Both the chance of serious complications from rubella infection (birth defects) and the chance of serious side effects from the vaccine (swelling of the joints) are very low. The severity of the consequences of a missed vaccine far outweighs that of receiving the vaccine. In addition, because rubella infections are usually without symptoms, the reported incidence of disease is far less than the actual incidence of infection. Decreased use of the vaccine will only increase the chance that pregnant women will be exposed to rubella and that rubella infection could damage their children.

Chapter 11

HEPATITIS B ("THE HEPATITIS VACCINE")

When William was only 12 hours old, his mother was handed a form by the nurse requesting permission to give him the Hep B vaccine.

Wasn't William too young to get a vaccine?

Why was it necessary to give him a vaccine when he was only 12 hours old?

The hepatitis B virus is one of a number of viruses that cause hepatitis (inflammation of the liver), cirrhosis (severe liver disease), and liver cancer. Every year about 300,000 people in the United States are infected with the hepatitis B virus.

Up until recently, the hepatitis B vaccine was recommended only for people at highest risk of acquiring hepatitis B virus infection (usually adolescents and young adults). This included health care workers, intravenous drug users, homosexuals, and people living in the house of someone infected with hepatitis B. Unfortunately, this policy didn't work, and the number of hepatitis B virus infections remained unchanged.

In 1991 a new policy was enacted: it was recommended that *all* infants receive the hepatitis B vaccine. Some parents feel that as their children will never be in a group at high risk of getting hepatitis B, they should not receive the vaccine. In this chapter we will discuss why the policy of immunizing all children makes sense.

Recommendation by the American Academy of Pediatrics

The American Academy of Pediatrics recommends that all infants and young children receive three doses of the hepatitis B vaccine. The first dose should be given between birth and 2 months of age; the second dose should be given one to two months after the first dose; and the third dose should be given between 6 months and 18 months of age.

WHAT IS HEPATITIS B?

Hepatitis B is a virus that infects the liver. Most children infected with the hepatitis B virus don't feel sick. A few children have a loss of appetite, tiredness, vomiting, nausea, and yellow eyes and skin (called jaundice).

The hepatitis B virus usually infects adolescents and young adults. Although most people get better, some carry the virus in their blood-stream for decades. These carriers may not look or feel sick, but they can spread the disease to other people.

WHAT IS THE HEPATITIS B VACCINE?

The hepatitis B virus is coated with hepatitis B surface protein. To be protected against the virus, you need immunity to this protein.

Researchers found a way to purify this protein and use it as a vaccine. Therefore, the hepatitis B vaccine does not contain hepatitis B virus—it contains only a small part of the virus coat.

The hepatitis B virus is unusual in that when it grows in liver cells, it makes more surface protein than it needs. Blood from infected people contains an excess of this surface protein, and this excess protein can be easily separated away from the infectious virus. In fact, there are about 50 trillion hepatitis B surface protein particles (not attached to infectious virus) in one teaspoon of blood. The first vaccine against hepatitis B took advantage of this phenomenon.

The first hepatitis B vaccine was made by taking blood from people infected with hepatitis B virus, treating it with chemicals that would kill any known infectious agent, and purifying the hepatitis B virus surface protein. The vaccine was used in this country from 1981 to 1992 and was both safe and effective.

Later, to relieve fears that the blood used to make the hepatitis B vaccine contained other infectious agents (such as the AIDS virus), a different approach was taken. Hepatitis B virus surface protein was manufactured by taking the gene that codes for the protein and inserting it into yeast cells. The surface protein made in the yeast cells was separated from them, purified, and used as a vaccine. This genetically engineered or "yeast-derived" vaccine was first introduced in the United States in 1986 and has proven to be both safe and effective. However, because of the way that it is made, the vaccine does contain small amounts of yeast cell proteins.

Is the hepatitis B vaccine safe?

More than 10 million adults and 2 million infants and children have been immunized in the United States, and at least 12 million children have been immunized worldwide. About 3 percent of children develop pain and tenderness where the shot was given; low-grade fevers occur in about 1 percent.

One extremely rare side effect of the hepatitis B vaccine is anaphylaxis (or hypersensitivity reaction). Symptoms of anaphylaxis include swelling of the mouth, breathing difficulties, low blood pressure, and shock. The incidence of anaphylaxis in children is estimated to be about one case per 600,000 doses given. Although it is a serious and frightening side effect, no one has ever died of anaphylaxis from the hepatitis B vaccine.

Because the vaccine is made in yeast cells, those with known allergies to yeast should not receive it.

Will the hepatitis B vaccine prevent my child from getting hepatitis?

Hepatitis is caused by several viruses. However, hepatitis B virus accounts for about 50 percent of all viral causes of hepatitis and is the most common cause of severe liver disease and liver cancer. Most of the other cases of viral hepatitis are caused by hepatitis A virus (for which there is also a vaccine; see Chapter 21).

So the hepatitis B vaccine does not prevent all cases of hepatitis, but it does prevent the most common cause of severe hepatitis.

Isn't hepatitis usually a mild infection?

Many people infected with hepatitis B never feel sick. However, each year in the United States 10,000 people are hospitalized and 400 die from liver damage caused by the virus.

In addition, carriers—people who carry hepatitis B virus in their blood for long periods of time—are likely to get severe liver disease (called cirrhosis) or liver cancer. There are currently more than 1 million carriers of hepatitis B virus in the United States. Four thousand carriers die from cirrhosis and 1,000 die from liver cancer every year.

The "Silent" Epidemic

"The existence of a worldwide pandemic can escape medical detection and public alarm when . . . its natural signs are obscure or separated in time by decades. Such was the case with hepatitis B. Its link to cancer and cirrhosis of the liver, sequelae that take thirty to forty years to appear . . . was entirely hidden. Thus, it was for thousands of years a 'silent' epidemic, whose dimensions and severity went undetected."

From William Muraskin's *The War Against Hepatitis B*, 1995.

How do you catch hepatitis B virus?

People infected with hepatitis B virus have large quantities of the virus in their blood. In fact, it is estimated that as many as 500 million infectious particles are present in about one teaspoon of blood from an infected person. The most likely way to catch hepatitis B virus is by coming in contact with small amounts of blood from an infected person.

Infants born to mothers who are infected with the hepatitis B virus are at high risk of getting the disease. During delivery, newborns come in contact with large quantities of blood in the birth canal. About 90 percent of newborns infected during delivery will not only be infected, but go on to develop chronic hepatitis B virus infection. Many of those with chronic infection will develop liver failure (cirrhosis) and die from the disease.

Others at risk of catching hepatitis B virus from infected people include intravenous drug users who share needles, health care workers exposed to blood, and sexual and family contacts of hepatitis B virus carriers. Because blood contains such a high quantity of infectious virus, family contacts are at risk simply by sharing washcloths, toothbrushes, razors, or nail clippers with an infected person.

The Hepatitis B Vaccine Is the Only Vaccine that Can Prevent Cancer

Hepatitis B virus is the second most common cause of cancer (specifically liver cancer) known to man.

Cigarette smoking is the first.

My son got the hepatitis B vaccine right after he was born. Isn't this too early to get a vaccine?

Newborns whose mothers are infected with the hepatitis B virus are exposed to large quantities of maternal blood at birth. Many of these children not only catch hepatitis B virus, but go on to develop chronic liver disease and die.

Every year in the United States, about 20,000 women give birth when they are infected with hepatitis B virus. By starting the series of vaccines within the first day of life, most infants born to mothers infected with the virus will be protected against hepatitis B infection.

What is most unusual about the hepatitis B vaccine is that it works even after newborns have been in contact with the virus. If newborns are exposed to maternal blood containing hepatitis B virus during delivery, then the virus may have a 24-hour head start on the vaccine. But the vaccine still works to prevent hepatitis B virus infections in these children. This is because the incubation period (the time from exposure to the virus to development of disease) for hepatitis B virus is fairly long (about 70 days on average).

Are the hep B shots that my daughter gets in her first year enough, or will she need more doses when she gets older?

The new hepatitis B vaccine has been around since 1986. There is no evidence that you need another dose beyond the series of three doses.

Why are all children supposed to get the hep B vaccine when only some of them are at risk?

Most people in the United States catch hepatitis B virus infection as adolescents or adults. People catch hepatitis B virus when they (1) have sexual contact with an infected person, (2) take care of an infected person in the hospital (for example, doctors, nurses, medical students, hemodialysis technicians), or (3) live in the home of someone infected with the virus.

Unfortunately, people who transmit the disease often don't know that they are infected with hepatitis B virus and are contagious. It is, therefore, very difficult to know for sure who is likely to get infected. Indeed, about 40 percent of people who catch hepatitis B virus have no idea where they got it from. For this reason, the strategy of selectively immunizing only people at highest risk didn't work in the United States. As a result, the vaccine has been recommended for all children in this country starting at birth.

My doctor tested my blood at the beginning of my pregnancy and said that I don't have hepatitis B. Why then does my baby have to get the hep B vaccine at birth?

Most pregnant women have blood taken to see whether they are infected with hepatitis B in the first trimester of pregnancy. However, hepatitis B virus is a common infection (about 300,000 cases a year), and many people are unaware of how they caught it. So women could become infected during the last two trimesters of pregnancy and pass the infection on to their babies. Because infection of infants with hepatitis B virus is often very severe and occasionally fatal, it is recommended that infants receive the vaccine at birth.

My 10-year-old daughter did not get the hep B vaccine during her routine shots. Should she get the vaccine now?

The recommendation that all infants born in this country receive the hepatitis B vaccine was made in 1991.

But what about those children who were born before we started to immunize all infants? Aren't they still at risk of getting hepatitis B when they become adolescents and adults? The answer to that question is obviously yes. Therefore, all children who didn't get the hepatitis B vaccine as infants should be immunized, preferably prior to adolescence (meaning by 11 to 12 years of age).

HEPATITIS B VACCINE: SUMMARY AND CONCLUSIONS

THE CHANCE OF CATCHING HEPATITIS B

There are about 300,000 people infected with the hepatitis B virus each year in the United States; of them, about 10,000 are hospitalized and 400 die from liver damage caused by the virus.

Infants born to mothers who are infected with hepatitis B virus are at great risk of getting infected during delivery and developing chronic hepatitis B virus infection.

The Risk of Serious Side Effects from the Hepatitis B Vaccine

A rare side effect of the hepatitis B vaccine is anaphylaxis, or hypersensitivity reaction. Symptoms of anaphylaxis include swelling of the mouth, breathing difficulties, low blood pressure, and shock. The incidence of anaphylaxis in children is estimated to be about one case per 600,000 doses given. Although a serious and frightening side effect, no one has ever died of anaphylaxis from the hepatitis B vaccine.

Conclusions

The incidence of severe and occasionally fatal hepatitis B virus infection in this country is still quite high. For this and other reasons, the hepatitis B vaccine is now recommended for routine use in all children.

Every year about 5,000 to 6,000 people die from hepatitis B virus infection. No one has ever died as a result of hepatitis B vaccination.

The benefits of giving the hepatitis B vaccine clearly outweigh the risks.

CHAPTER 12

VARICELLA ("THE CHICKENPOX VACCINE")

Rebecca is 1 year old. Her mother takes her to the doctor and finds out that there is a new vaccine, called the varicella vaccine, that prevents chickenpox.

The doctor tells Rebecca's mother that chickenpox is usually a mild disease and that she can decide whether Rebecca should be immunized. Rebecca's mother has some friends whose children have gotten the vaccine and some whose children haven't.

Should Rebecca get the chickenpox vaccine?

The varicella vaccine was approved for use in children in 1995. Since then it has gradually attained widespread acceptance.

Despite acceptance by most parents and doctors, a number of questions about the varicella vaccine have been raised:

1. Why prevent a disease as mild as chickenpox?
2. If children are immunized, won't the disease just occur more frequently in adults?
3. Can the chickenpox vaccine cause shingles?
4. Can adults or other children catch chickenpox from someone given the varicella vaccine?

In this chapter we will address each of these questions.

Recommendation by the American Academy of Pediatrics

In March of 1995 the Food and Drug Administration licensed the varicella vaccine, and in May of 1995 the American Academy of Pediatrics recommended its use for children. The varicella vaccine should be given as a single shot between 1 and 12 years of age to children who have not previously had chickenpox.

WHAT IS CHICKENPOX?

. . . Measles makes you bumpy,

and mumps will make you lumpy,

and chickenpox will make you jump and twitch. . . .

From "Poison Ivy" by The Coasters, 1959.

Chickenpox is an infection caused by the varicella virus. The infection usually starts as a rash on the face that spreads to the rest of the body. The rash begins as red bumps that eventually become blisters—a child often will get 300 to 500 blisters during a single infection. The blisters eventually "crust over" and fall off in one to two weeks.

Each year there are 3 to 4 million cases of chickenpox in the United States. Most cases occur in children younger than 10 years old.

WHAT IS THE CHICKENPOX VACCINE?

The varicella virus normally grows in cells that line the back of child's throat and in skin cells. The varicella vaccine was made by taking varicella virus from one of the blisters of an infected child in Japan (the family name of the child was Oka, and the strain of virus in the vaccine is called the Oka strain). The virus was then grown in several specialized cells in the laboratory. The cells in which the varicella virus vaccine was grown included both human and guinea pig fibroblast cells (fibroblasts are cells that help hold tissues together). As the varicella virus became better and better able to grow in these fibroblast cells, it became less and less able to grow in a child's skin or throat. When this cell-culture–adapted virus (the vaccine virus) was given to children, it replicated only a little before it was eliminated from the body.

The varicella vaccine is a live, weakened (or attenuated) virus.

Is the chickenpox vaccine safe?

About 20 percent of children given the varicella vaccine will have pain where the shot was administered. About 10 percent will have low-grade fever.

A rash caused by the varicella vaccine occurs in about 4 percent of vaccinated children. Some will develop a rash where the shot was given, and some will get a generalized rash. On average, when a rash does occur, the number of blisters from the vaccine is about ten.

The varicella vaccine causes this mild rash because it is still a live virus. However, the vaccine virus is so weak that it is not efficiently transferred from someone who got the vaccine to another person. Therefore, the varicella vaccine can be given even to those children who are living in the home of someone whose immune system is weak (for example, family members with leukemia, lymphoma, or other types of cancers). The vaccine can also be given to children whose mother is pregnant.

Why should we prevent a disease as mild as chickenpox?

Although chickenpox is very uncomfortable, most children recover without difficulty. For some children, however, chickenpox can have disastrous consequences. For example, about one out of every thousand children infected with chickenpox will develop severe pneumonia or infection of the brain (encephalitis).

Varicella can also cause birth defects. Birth defects occur in about 2 percent of children born to women infected during their pregnancy and include severe scarring of the skin, shortened limbs, mental retardation, and cataracts.

In addition, varicella has been increasingly associated with skin infections caused by a dangerous bacterium called Group A B-hemolytic streptococcus. This particular bacterium, popularized in the media as the "flesh-eating" bacterium, can cause severe and fatal infections.

Although not often mentioned as a complication of chickenpox infection, many children are left with permanent facial scars caused by varicella blisters.

At least 9,000 people are hospitalized and 100 die of chickenpox each year in the United States. Almost all of the hospitalizations and deaths from this infection occur in previously healthy young children.

Chickenpox Should Not Be a Childhood "Rite of Passage"

Complications from Chickenpox Each Year	
Hospitalizations	9,000
Pneumonia	4,000
Brain infection	600
Deaths	100

A TRUE STORY

The mother of a healthy 8-year-old girl took her to the doctor for a physical required for camp. The mother had heard about the chickenpox vaccine and asked her doctor about it. The doctor explained that chickenpox was usually a mild infection and that he didn't feel strongly about the vaccine one way or the other. The mother chose not to give her daughter the vaccine.

Six months later the child developed chickenpox, with a blistering rash and fever. Over the course of several days, she had progressive difficulty breathing and was eventually taken to the Emergency Department. A chest X ray showed that the child had pneumonia caused by varicella. She was admitted to the hospital.

Over the next two days the girl developed more difficulty breathing and had to be intubated and put on a respirator. A new chest X ray showed that she had developed a bacterial pneumonia on top of what was already a varicella pneumonia. Fluid taken from the child's lung showed that the bacteria was Group A B-hemolytic strep. (These bacteria, popularly referred to as "flesh-eating" bacteria, are occasionally associated with chickenpox.)

The child was in the intensive care unit for two weeks but survived.

If we immunize children, will they be more likely to get chickenpox as adults?

Like many viral infections, including measles, mumps, and rubella, chickenpox is more severe in adults than in children. Adults with chickenpox are more likely to develop severe pneumonia or encephalitis than are children. As a consequence, they are 15 times more likely than children to die from chickenpox. Therefore, it is extremely important to try to prevent adults from getting chickenpox.

Our experience with the measles, mumps, and rubella vaccines has taught us that fading immunity after immunization shouldn't be a problem with the varicella vaccine. All three of these diseases were more common in children than adults before their vaccines were developed. After children were immunized with the combination of measles, mumps, and rubella vaccines, the incidence of these diseases decreased dramatically not only in children but also in adults. In addition, the varicella vaccine has been used in children in Japan for about 20 years without any evidence of fading immunity.

Can the chickenpox vaccine cause shingles?

Shingles is a rash with extremely painful and disfiguring blisters on the face, chest, or abdomen. There are about 300,000 cases of shingles in the United States each year; most occur in elderly adults.

Shingles occurs only in people who have already had chickenpox. After recovery from chickenpox, varicella virus lives silently in the nervous system. As we age, it becomes more and more likely that the virus will reawaken, or reactivate, and infect the skin.

You can get shingles after either chickenpox infection or varicella vaccine. However, shingles after the vaccine is much less frequent and much less severe than after chickenpox.

The Varicella Vaccine Will Probably Prevent Shingles, Too

After chickenpox infection, varicella virus travels from the skin to the nervous system, where it lives silently (or latently) for many years. As we get older, the virus reawakens, or reactivates, and infects the nerves and skin in a condition called shingles. Shingles is incredibly painful and debilitating. Blisters can occur on the face or in the eye and last for several weeks. In addition, shingles is quite common—up to 20 percent of adults will have had it by the time they are 80 years old.

After immunization with varicella vaccine, the virus also probably travels to the nervous system, where it lives latently. But because the vaccine virus is much less likely to cause a rash than the natural (or "wild-type" virus) infection, there is probably less vaccine virus than natural virus traveling to the nervous tissue.

The key question is which of these two viruses you would rather have living in your nervous system: "wild-type" virus, which is well adapted to growth in nervous tissue, or the weakened vaccine virus, which is not.

All the evidence gathered over the last 20 years has shown just what you would expect. "Wild-type" varicella virus reactivates more frequently and causes more severe shingles than vaccine virus.

I'm afraid to try a vaccine that is so new. Shouldn't I wait until the vaccine has been around for a while before I use it?

The varicella vaccine has been tested in children since the early 1970s. There were 20 years of experience with the vaccine before it was licensed in the United States—about five times more experience than any other vaccine had before licensure.

VARICELLA VACCINE: SUMMARY AND CONCLUSIONS

THE CHANCE OF CATCHING CHICKENPOX

The varicella vaccine was only recently licensed in this country (in March 1995). At the time of licensure, there were about 3 to 4 million cases of chickenpox infection every year in the United States.

Chickenpox is usually an uncomfortable infection characterized by fever and about 300 to 500 blisters. Most children recover from the infection without problems. However, for some, chickenpox can have disastrous consequences. For example, about one out of every thousand children infected with chickenpox will develop severe pneumonia or infection of the brain (encephalitis).

Chickenpox also causes birth defects in about 2 percent of children born to women infected during their pregnancy. These birth defects include severe scarring of the skin, shortened limbs, mental retardation, and cataracts.

At least 9,000 people are hospitalized and 100 die of chickenpox each year in the United States. Most of these hospitalizations and deaths occur in previously healthy children.

THE RISK OF SERIOUS SIDE EFFECTS FROM THE VARICELLA VACCINE

The varicella vaccine has been given to children for over 20 years. There are no serious side effects from the vaccine.

Although it is likely to live silently in the nervous system of vaccinated children, there is no evidence that the vaccine virus is more dangerous than the natural virus. In fact, all evidence to date shows that the vaccine virus is weaker than the natural virus and therefore less likely to cause shingles when the virus awakens, or reactivates.

Conclusions

Because chickenpox is still prevalent in this country, parents choosing not to get the vaccine are in effect choosing natural or "wild-type" virus infection for their children. Most children will survive this infection without any problems, but chickenpox is a rare cause of permanent disability and death.

The benefits of the varicella vaccine clearly outweigh the risks.

CHAPTER 1 3

PRACTICAL TIPS ABOUT VACCINES

FEAR OF SHOTS

Many children are afraid to go to the doctor's office when they know it's time to get shots. There are, however, some techniques that can help children through this occasionally frightening experience.

Gina French and her coworkers at The Children's Hospital in Columbus, Ohio, published a study evaluating the capacity of breathing techniques to ease the pain caused by immunizations. Their study was called "Blowing Away Shot Pain." They studied about 150 children between 4 and 7 years of age who were about to be immunized. Half of the children were treated as usual. The other half were told the following: "I know a trick that might make it easier. It is something that children who get lots of shots use. When it is time for the shot you should take a deep breath and blow and blow and blow until I tell you to stop." The child was then asked to practice this technique with the investigator. After the shots were given, the children were asked to evaluate their pain on a scale from "no hurt at all" to "the worst in the world."

Children who had been coached in the breathing techniques rated their pain as significantly less than those who hadn't.

WHO SHOULDN'T GET VACCINES

Any child who has had a severe reaction to a vaccine should not receive another dose of that same vaccine. Severe reactions include difficulty breathing, hives, low blood pressure, or shock and usually occur immediately after receiving the shot.

Also, the live, weakened vaccines should not be given to children with leukemia, lymphoma, other types of cancers, or AIDS. The live, weakened vaccine viruses include measles, mumps, rubella, varicella, and oral polio (OPV).

VACCINATING CHILDREN WHO LIVE WITH SOMEONE WITH WEAKENED IMMUNITY

Children living in the home with someone who has weakened immunity (such as leukemia, lymphoma, or other types of cancers) should not receive vaccines that are potentially contagious.

The oral polio virus vaccine (OPV) is found in the intestines of vaccinated children in high quantities, and children immunized with OPV are definitely contagious. Therefore, the oral polio vaccine should not be given to healthy children living in a home with an adult or child with weakened immunity. These children should get the inactivated polio vaccine (IPV) instead for all four doses.

Live virus vaccines such as measles, mumps, rubella, and varicella can occasionally be found in the throat of vaccinated children. However, because these vaccine viruses are weakened, and because they are detected in such low amounts, children who are immunized with them are rarely, if ever, contagious. Therefore, children living in a home with someone with weakened immunity can get the measles, mumps, rubella, and varicella vaccines.

Children who receive vaccines that contain only a part of a virus or bacterium (hepatitis B, Hib, DTaP) or a killed virus (IPV) are not contagious.

VACCINATING CHILDREN WHO ARE ILL

Unfortunately, illness is a common reason for many children to miss vaccines. It is safe to give all of the recommended vaccines to children with minor illnesses. Minor illnesses include low-grade fever, ear infections, cough, runny nose, diarrhea, or vomiting.

PREGNANCY

Sometimes infants and toddlers are supposed to receive vaccines at the same time that their mother is pregnant.

The only vaccine that can be contagious to the pregnant mother is the oral polio vaccine (OPV). Since polio virus doesn't infect the unborn child, this vaccine is safe to give to a child whose mother is pregnant. Children who receive the other live, weakened virus vaccines (measles, mumps, rubella, or varicella) are not likely to be contagious. Therefore, a child with a pregnant mother may receive *all* the recommended vaccines.

BREAST-FEEDING

It is unlikely that the antibodies found in breast milk can interfere with the ability of vaccines to induce protective immunity in infants. Therefore, all infants who are breast-feeding may receive all the recommended vaccines.

STEROIDS

Steroids are occasionally given to children with common diseases such as asthma or poison ivy. Because steroids can weaken the immune system, parents ask whether it is safe to give vaccines at the same time children are getting steroids.

The answer is yes and no. It is safe for children who have received steroid creams or steroid sprays (aerosols) to get vaccines. Vaccines are also safe for children who have received steroids by mouth for less than two weeks. However, children who have received high doses of steroids (meaning more than 2 mg/kg per day of prednisone or its equivalent) by mouth for more than two weeks should *not* receive live, weakened virus vaccines (specifically, measles, mumps, rubella, varicella, or oral polio). High doses of steroids may decrease a child's ability to fight infection, as well as the ability to build immunity after vaccination.

ANTIBIOTIC ALLERGIES

Some children have severe allergic reactions to antibiotics. These reactions may include hives, difficulty breathing, low blood pressure, or shock.

None of the vaccines contain antibiotics to which children are usually allergic (such as penicillins and cephalosporins). Some vaccines contain trace amounts of antibiotics that are extremely rare causes of allergic reactions and to which most children have never been exposed (specifically, neomycin and streptomycin).

Therefore, children allergic to penicillin, amoxicillin, cephalosporins, or sulfa drugs may receive all the recommended vaccines.

EGG ALLERGIES

Some children are highly allergic to the proteins in eggs. Allergic reactions include hives, difficulty breathing, and shock.

Both the measles and mumps vaccines are made in cells originally derived from chick eggs. However, there are not enough chicken proteins in the final vaccine preparation to cause problems. Recent studies have shown that even children with severe egg allergies can receive these vaccines without difficulty.

Children with severe egg allergies should not, however, receive either the influenza or yellow fever vaccines.

VACCINATING PREMATURE BABIES

Most premature infants, including those with low birth weights, can be immunized at the usual chronological age. In other words, a child born two months early should still receive his or her first immunization at 2 months of age (not at 4 months of age).

The only exception to this rule is the hepatitis B vaccine. Premature infants (children born within 36 weeks' gestation with a birth weight of less than 4.4 pounds) whose mothers are not infected with the hepatitis B virus should receive the hepatitis B vaccine at two months of age rather than at birth. However, premature infants whose mothers *are* infected with the hepatitis B virus should receive the vaccine at birth, independent of birth weight.

SIMULTANEOUS VACCINES

Because of the new varicella, hepatitis B, and pertussis vaccines, some children will receive as many as three or four vaccines during a single visit to the pediatrician. This is obviously frightening for children and parents and cumbersome for the doctor. The good news is that several vaccine manufacturers are working on making combination vaccines to reduce the number of shots (see Chapter 27).

All routinely recommended vaccines can be given simultaneously. There is no evidence that giving one vaccine significantly interferes with the immunity caused by another. Nor is there evidence that any of the vaccines increases the rate of side effects of another. Different vaccines should, however, be given at different sites of the body.

MISSED VACCINES

A missed vaccine does not mean that the series must be started all over again. If a dose of DTaP, oral polio (OPV), Hib, or hepatitis B vaccine is missed, the series of immunizations can be continued after the missing dose(s) is given.

VACCINATING CHILDREN ADOPTED FROM OTHER COUNTRIES

Children vaccinated in other countries should be immunized according to the same schedule as that required for children in the United States. However, only a written record of immunization should be accepted as evidence that a child has been vaccinated either in this country or elsewhere. The majority of vaccines made in other parts of the world, including developing countries, are produced with adequate quality control standards and are of reliable potency.

CHAPTER 14

THE GREAT
VACCINE MYTHS

It seems that almost every month there are newspaper articles and television programs depicting the horrors of vaccines. The villains are greedy vaccine manufacturers, disinterested doctors, and burdensome regulatory agencies. The focus of the stories is that children are hurt unnecessarily by vaccines, and the tone is one of intrigue and cover-up.

Perhaps the most dangerous part of these stories (apart from the fact that they may cause many children to miss the vaccines they need) is that the science is presented in a manner that seems believable. Below we have listed the most commonly aired stories about vaccines and have tried to separate fact from myth.

MYTH: Vaccines don't work.

Probably the best example of the impact of vaccines is the Hib vaccine, a vaccine that prevents meningitis caused by the bacterium *Haemophilus influenzae type b* (Hib).

The current Hib vaccine was first introduced to this country in 1990. At that time, Hib was the most common cause of bacterial meningitis, accounting for approximately 8,000 cases and 400 to 500 deaths every year. The incidence of cases and deaths per year had been steady for decades. After the current Hib vaccine was introduced, the incidence of Hib meningitis declined to fewer than 50 cases per year.

The power of the Hib vaccine is that all pediatricians and family practitioners working today saw its impact.

MYTH: Vaccines are not safe.

Despite what is often stated in the media, all recommended vaccines are extraordinarily safe. Side effects from vaccines are usually limited to pain and tenderness where the shot was given or low-grade fever.

However, side effects from two vaccines are more worrisome: the "old" pertussis vaccine and the oral polio vaccine (OPV) (see Chapters 7 and 8 for more details). The "old" pertussis vaccine (in the preparation called DTP) was a rare cause of persistent crying, seizures, and high fever. Although children were not permanently damaged by the vaccine, it was still very difficult for parents to watch their children suffer these side effects. Fortunately, the new pertussis vaccine (DTaP) is purer than the old vaccine and will virtually eliminate these rare side effects.

The other vaccine that is problematic is oral polio vaccine. OPV itself can be a rare cause of complete and lifelong paralysis, usually after the first dose. Because the polio virus was eliminated from the Western Hemisphere in 1991, the only children who now get polio in this country are those who received OPV. We support the new recommendation by the Centers for Disease Control and Prevention that the first two doses of the polio vaccine be with the inactivated vaccine, or IPV. This change in policy will help eliminate this rare but devastating side effect.

MYTH: Infants are too young to get vaccinated.

Children are immunized in the first few months of life because a number of vaccine-preventable diseases infect them when they are very young.

For example:

- Pertussis infects 3,000 children, causing six deaths every year in the United States. Almost all of the cases are in children *less than 1 year of age.*

- Children *under 2 years old* are 500 times more likely to catch Hib meningitis if someone with a Hib infection is living in the home.

- About 90 percent of *newborns* whose mothers are infected with hepatitis B will contract hepatitis.

For these reasons, it is very important for infants to be fully immunized against certain diseases by the time they are 6 months old.

Fortunately, young infants are surprisingly good at building immunity to viruses and bacteria. About 95 percent of children given DTaP, Hib, and hepatitis B virus vaccines will be fully protected by 6 months of age.

MYTH: It's better to be naturally infected than immunized.

It is true that "natural" infection almost always causes better immunity than vaccination (only the Hib and tetanus vaccines are better at inducing immunity than natural infection). Whereas natural infection causes immunity after just one infection, vaccines usually create immunity only after several doses are given over a number of years. For example, DTaP, hepatitis B, and polio are each given at least three times.

However, the difference between vaccination and natural infection is the price paid for immunity (see Chapter 2). The price paid for vaccination is the inconvenience of several shots and the occasional sore arm. The price paid for a single natural infection can be considerably greater. Paralysis from natural polio infection, meningitis from natural Hib infection, liver failure from natural hepatitis B virus infection, deafness from natural mumps infection, or pneumonia from natural varicella infection are high prices to pay for immunity.

MYTH: Vaccines weaken the immune system.

Certain viruses can indeed weaken the immune system. This means that when children are infected with one virus, they can't fight off other viruses or bacteria as easily. This happens most notably during infection with either chickenpox or measles.

But vaccines are different. The viruses in the measles and chickenpox vaccines (the so-called vaccine viruses) are very different from those that cause measles and chickenpox infections (the "wild-type" viruses). The vaccine viruses are themselves so disabled that they cannot weaken the immune system.

MYTH: Vaccines use up the immune system.

Is it possible that all the vaccines given to children in the first few months of life use up the immune system? Certainly children build immunity to only a limited number of microorganisms (viruses, bacteria, fungi, or parasites). The question is, how many?

Probably the most sensible approach to answering this question was that formulated by Drs. Mel Cohn and Rodney Langman, immunologists working at the Developmental Biology Laboratory at The Salk Institute in San Diego. They theorized that the number of microorganisms to which a body can respond depends on the number of cells in blood that can make antibodies sufficient to recognize all the relevant parts of the microorganism.

Using their theory (called the Protecton Theory), it stood to reason that the number of microorganisms to which one responds depends on one's size. Cohn and Langman estimated that elephants can produce immunity to about 100 times more organisms than humans, and that humans can build immunity to at least 100 times more organisms than hummingbirds. Although this would mean that adult humans can make antibodies to more organisms than infants, the scientists estimated that humans can respond to about 100,000 different organisms.

Therefore, the ten vaccines required for all children will use up only about 0.01 percent of the immunity that is available.

MYTH: *Some vaccines contain other infectious agents that may damage my child.*

All currently recommended vaccines are tested by pharmaceutical companies under the strict supervision of the Food and Drug Administration (FDA). Vaccines are tested for the presence of known viruses, bacteria, fungi, or parasites different from those contained in the vaccine.

When you consider that the 3.5 to 4 million children born every year in the United States receive ten different vaccines by the time they are 6 years old, and that some of these vaccines have been in existence for over 50 years, the record of vaccine safety in this country is remarkable.

MYTH: *The DTP vaccine caused deafness in the winner of the Miss America pageant in 1994.*

The Miss America winner was supposedly rendered permanently deaf by a bad DTP vaccine—a story that got a lot of play in the news media in 1994. These reports were totally false. Overlooked was the fact her deafness followed a case of bacterial meningitis as a child. The cause of the meningitis was *Haemophilus influenzae type b* (Hib), a bacterium for which a vaccine became available in this country in 1990. Hib meningitis caused deafness in up to 20 percent of children in the past. Fortunately, the Hib vaccine has virtually eliminated Hib meningitis.

MYTH: *The polio vaccine is the cause of AIDS.*

Tom Curtis wrote an article in *Rolling Stone* magazine claiming that the origin of AIDS could be traced to polio virus vaccines that were administered in the Belgian Congo between 1957 and 1960. The logic behind this assertion was as follows: (1) All virus vaccines are made in cells, (2) the poliovirus vaccine was grown in monkey kidney cells, (3) monkey kidney cells used at that time contained a virus (simian immunodeficiency virus, or SIV) similar to the virus that causes AIDS (human immunodeficiency virus, or HIV), and (4) people were inadvertently inoculated with SIV, which then mutated to HIV and caused the AIDS epidemic.

There are many problems with this reasoning. First, although monkeys can be infected by SIV, a disease similar to HIV, SIV is not found in kidney cells. Second, SIV and HIV, although their spelling is very similar, are not genetically very close; mutation to one from the other would require centuries, not years. Third, SIV and HIV, although deadly viruses, are fairly fragile. Both of these viruses, if given by mouth (in a manner similar to the oral polio vaccine), would be rapidly destroyed by the enzymes and acids in the mouth and stomach. Lastly, original lots of the polio vaccine were recently tested for the presence of HIV using very sensitive tests that were not available in the late 1950s. These tests, called polymerase chain reaction, or PCR, are used today to diagnose HIV infection in children, adolescents, and adults. No HIV was present in any of those lots.

MYTH: The polio virus vaccine is contaminated with a virus that causes cancer.

It is true that early lots of the poliovirus vaccine used in the late 1950s and early 1960s were contaminated with a monkey virus called simian virus 40, or SV40. Recently "tracks" of SV40 have been identified by researchers in unusual tumors in adults. The studies have been suggestive enough that the National Institutes of Health are monitoring ongoing research for a possible link.

However, none of the currently manufactured polio vaccines—neither the live vaccine given by mouth (OPV) nor the killed vaccine given as a shot (IPV) contain SV40. Therefore, current poliovirus vaccines pose no risk of coming in contact with SV40.

MYTH: The pertussis vaccine doesn't work. The incidence of pertussis was declining before we used pertussis vaccine in the United States.

The pertussis vaccine was introduced into the United States in the mid-1940s. Between 1900 and 1940, the incidence of pertussis was definitely declining. This decline was due to improved hygiene and sanitation.

However, the pertussis vaccine hastened the decline of the disease. There are five pieces of evidence that prove the vaccine's efficacy:

- In clinical trials of the pertussis vaccine, those who received the vaccine were protected against pertussis, whereas those who didn't receive it were not.

- Introduction of the pertussis vaccine into communities leads to a rapid decline in the incidence of pertussis.

- Pertussis recurs in countries in which the vaccine has been discontinued or immunization rates have declined.

- In communities where pertussis is always around (i.e., is endemic), the incidence of disease is inversely correlated with the percentage of children immunized.

- When epidemics of pertussis occur, unimmunized children are more likely to get pertussis than immunized children.

PART THREE

VACCINES FOR SOME CHILDREN

CHAPTER 15

RABIES

Katherine is 7 years old. While playing in the backyard of a friend's house she is bitten on the hand by a cat. None of her friends ever saw the cat before, and it has not been seen since.

Should Katherine get the rabies vaccine?

Rabies is a uniformly fatal infection that is transmitted to children by the bite of a rabies-infected, or rabid, animal. Because children are occasionally bitten or scratched by animals, physicians and parents are commonly forced to decide about beginning a series of rabies shots.

The decision of whether to start this series of shots is a difficult one. Fortunately, however, it's not as hard as it used to be. Before 1980, rabies immunization meant a series of up to 30 shots given in the skin over the abdomen. This was often a painful and frightening experience for children and parents. Also, the vaccine didn't always work. About 20 percent of those immunized consists of still not protected against rabies.

Today rabies immunization consists of a series of five shots given in the shoulder muscle, and the vaccine is completely protective and very safe. In this chapter we will talk about who should get the rabies vaccine and why.

Recommendation by the American Academy of Pediatrics

Treatment of children bitten by an animal likely to transmit rabies consists of the following three things:

1. Washing the wound carefully with soap and water.
2. Rabies immune globulin.
3. Rabies vaccine at the time of exposure and then 3, 7, 14, and 28 days after exposure (a total of five shots). Shots are given in the shoulder muscle.

WHAT IS RABIES?

Rabies is a virus that infects the brain and nervous system and, because virtually no one survives infection, is one of the most feared diseases. It is transmitted to humans from the bite of an infected animal.

The disease usually begins with indistinct symptoms such as fatigue, sore throat, chills, vomiting, and headache. After about one week, symptoms may include hallucinations, bizarre behavior, disorientation, hyperactivity, and the inability to swallow. Progression to paralysis, coma, and death is inevitable.

Although cases of rabies in developed countries have received intensive medical support, only three people are known to have ever survived the infection.

Rabies Vaccine Works Even *After* Exposure to Rabies

The rabies vaccine is unusual in that it works even after someone is infected with the virus. Rabies has a long incubation period (the time from exposure to development of symptoms). Whereas diseases such as influenza have incubation periods as short as one or two days, the average incubation period for rabies is about two months. This means that after a bite from an infected animal there is still plenty of time (before symptoms appear) to develop protective immunity.

WHAT IS THE RABIES VACCINE?

The rabies virus normally grows in cells of the human nervous system. The rabies vaccine was made by taking rabies virus from the nervous system of an infected person and adapting it to growth in specialized cells grown in the laboratory. The cells in which rabies virus was grown were human lung cells (the vaccine is also called the human diploid cell vaccine, or HDCV). To make a vaccine, rabies virus was grown in these cells, purified, and inactivated with a chemical (B-propiolactone). Because the rabies virus can't replicate, it is called a killed, or inactivated, vaccine.

More than 500 people bitten by animals proven to be infected with rabies have received rabies vaccine (HDCV). None of these people got rabies. Therefore, the vaccine, if used correctly, appears to be 100 percent effective.

The First Rabies Vaccine

The rabies vaccine was developed by Louis Pasteur in the late 19th century. An account of the first child to receive the vaccine follows:

"Mrs. Meister from Meissnegott in Alsace . . . came crying into the laboratory, leading her 9-year-old boy, Joseph, gashed in fourteen places two days before by a mad dog. He was a pitifully whimpering, scared boy—hardly able to walk.

"'Save my little boy—Mr. Pasteur,' this woman begged him. . . .

"And that night of July 6, 1885, they made the first injection of the weakened microbes of hydrophobia [rabies] into a human being. Then, day after day, the boy Meister went without a hitch through his fourteen injections—which were only slight pricks of the hypodermic needle into his skin.

"And the boy went home to Alsace and had never a sign of that dreadful disease."

From Paul de Kruif's *Microbe Hunters*, 1926.

Doesn't the rabies vaccine mean getting many painful shots?

The rabies vaccine used in this country until 1980 had some problems. The virus was grown in cells from duck eggs (called duck embryo vaccine, or DEV) and had a fairly high rate of side effects.

The DEV was given as a series of from 23 to 30 shots in the skin over the abdomen. Even after this torturous experience, up to 20 percent of children were not protected against rabies. The DEV is no longer available in the United States and has been replaced by HDCV.

Who should get the rabies vaccine?

The rabies vaccine should be given to any child who is exposed to an animal likely to have rabies.

What counts as an exposure?

Rabies can be transmitted by a bite or a nonbite exposure from a rabid animal. A bite means that the animal's teeth have penetrated the child's skin. A nonbite means that a rabid animal has licked an open wound, a scratch, a cut, or a mucous membrane (such as the mouth, nose, or eyes). Therefore, neither petting a rabid animal nor getting scratched by an animal that does not break the skin would be considered an exposure.

What animals are likely to have rabies?

The animals likely to have rabies are determined by the area in which you live. Therefore, the smartest thing a parent can do after an animal bite is to call the local health department and find out whether a particular species of animal in that area is likely to be rabid. There are a few general rules that can be reassuring in the meantime:

1. Because most dogs and cats in the United States get a rabies vaccine, it is uncommon for them to catch or transmit rabies. If a child is bitten by a dog or cat, the animal should be observed for ten days. If the animal acts normally (doesn't show signs of rabies), there is no need for the vaccine. If the animal cannot be observed, then the vaccine should begin as outlined above.

2. Animals such as mice, rats, squirrels, rabbits, birds, chipmunks, or reptiles rarely, if ever, transmit rabies.

3. The animals most likely to transmit rabies in the United States are raccoons, skunks, foxes, and bats. Treatment should usually be given after bites from any of these animals.

Is the rabies vaccine safe?

More than 1 million doses of the HDCV rabies vaccine have been given, and the vaccine is safe. Even infants may receive it, if necessary.

However, the vaccine does have a fairly high rate of *mild* side effects. Some people who receive the rabies vaccine develop a sore arm (15 to 25 percent), headache (5 to 8 percent), or nausea (2 to 5 percent).

The HDCV rabies vaccine is also associated with allergic reactions. After the first dose, there have been several reported cases of anaphylaxis characterized by swelling of the mouth or throat, low blood pressure, or hives (0.1 percent). In addition, the incidence of anaphylaxis from subsequent, or booster, doses of the rabies vaccine can be as high as 6 percent. There has not been a fatality caused by the HDCV rabies vaccine.

Can you get rabies from the rabies vaccine?

Because the rabies virus in the vaccine is inactivated, it is not possible to get rabies from the vaccine.

RABIES VACCINE: SUMMARY AND CONCLUSIONS

Rabies is caused by a virus transmitted by the bite of a rabid animal. Because children are occasionally bitten or scratched by animals potentially infected with rabies, parents and physicians are confronted with the decision of whether to begin the series of rabies shots. Before 1980, the decision of whether to begin a series of rabies shots was hard; the "old" vaccine involved a series of 23 to 30 shots, didn't always work, and had a fairly high rate of side effects. These days the decision is easier; the current rabies vaccine is safe, is virtually 100 percent effective, and involves a series of only five shots.

CHAPTER 16

INFLUENZA ("THE FLU VACCINE")

Sarah is 3 years old. It seems that every time she gets a cold she wheezes. About six months ago, Sarah had an episode in which the wheezing was so bad that she had to see the doctor in the emergency room. The doctor says that Sarah has asthma and that she will probably grow out of it.

Sarah's mother has heard that children who have asthma may benefit from getting the influenza vaccine. Is this true?

Influenza, or flu, is a highly contagious viral illness that causes high fever, muscle aches, and coughing. Some children are at risk of getting severe or fatal pneumonia from influenza.

Children at risk of contracting severe influenza disease should get the influenza vaccine. For example, the vaccine is recommended for use in all children with asthma. Further, the influenza vaccine should be given to parents and siblings living in the home of someone with asthma. Because the vaccine is not often given to those who really need it, it is probably the most underused vaccine in pediatrics.

The influenza vaccine is unusual in that it is given every year. This is because the influenza viruses that cause disease one year are often different from those that cause it the following year.

In this chapter we will discuss who should get the influenza vaccine and why.

Recommendation by the American Academy of Pediatrics

The American Academy of Pediatrics recommends that children older than 6 months of age who are at risk for severe influenza infection (see the list below) should receive the influenza vaccine *every fall*. If the child is receiving influenza vaccine for the first time and is between 6 months and 8 years of age, the vaccine is given as two shots one month apart. If the child is 9 years old or older, the first dose of the vaccine is given as a single shot.

All subsequent, yearly doses of vaccine are given as a single shot.

WHAT IS INFLUENZA?

Influenza, or flu, is a virus that infects the windpipe (the trachea) and breathing tubes (bronchi). It usually begins with high fever, chills, severe muscle aches, and headache. These symptoms are so severe that patients usually remember the exact hour when the illness began.

As the fever and muscle aches subside, the patient develops a runny nose, cough, and sometimes a feeling of burning in the chest. These symptoms are caused by the destruction of the lining of the trachea and bronchi. The cough can last as long as one to two weeks.

Up to 25 percent of people develop complications from influenza. These complications include severe pneumonia or worsening of asthma.

Influenza Causes Epidemics and Pandemics

Epidemics are outbreaks of an infection confined to a specific location (such as a town, city, or country). Influenza epidemics occur every one to three years in the United States and kill about 10,000 people yearly.

Each century, influenza causes about eight pandemics (outbreaks of disease that occur worldwide). The worst pandemic in recent history occurred between 1918 and 1919, when 550,000 people were killed in the United States and 21 million people were killed throughout the world by influenza.

WHAT IS THE INFLUENZA VACCINE?

The influenza virus normally grows in cells that line the windpipe (trachea) and breathing tubes (bronchi). The influenza vaccine is made by taking influenza viruses from the throats of infected children and adapting them to growth in chicken embryos. The virus is then harvested from the eggs, purified, and inactivated with formaldehyde. The vaccine contains the three strains of influenza that are likely to cause infection that year.

Because the influenza virus in the vaccine cannot replicate, it is called a killed, or inactivated, vaccine.

The Great Epidemic

"By December of that year of mingled victory and catastrophe, 1918, five hundred thousand Americans had perished in a great plague, and nearly 20 million had sickened. The world had never in history been ravaged by a killer that slew so many human beings so quickly, during a few weeks in autumn.

"This microscopic marauder that could not be seen, heard, or even sensed, and was infinitely more deadly than any weapon from the crucible of the World War, was labeled, almost beguilingly, 'Spanish influenza.'"

From A. A. Hoehling, *The Great Epidemic*, 1961.

Is the influenza vaccine safe?

Fever, muscle aches, and malaise occur in less than 1 percent of those who receive the influenza vaccine. These side effects usually begin six to twelve hours after vaccination and can persist for one to two days. Side effects are most likely to occur in those who were never before infected with influenza virus or never immunized with influenza vaccine (usually younger children).

Sometimes people who have symptoms of fever, muscle aches, and malaise claim that they "got the flu" from the influenza vaccine. However, because the influenza virus in the vaccine is inactivated, it cannot cause the respiratory symptoms or pneumonia commonly seen in influenza infections.

In rare instances, immediate allergic reactions (hives, asthma, swelling of the throat, low blood pressure, or shock) occur after getting the influenza vaccine. These reactions are probably caused by allergies to the residual egg proteins in the vaccine. For this reason, *people with severe allergy to eggs are generally advised not to receive the influenza vaccine.* However, for those people who are at great risk for severe influenza disease (such as children with asthma), there are methods to desensitize the person to the vaccine prior to administration.

Who should get the influenza vaccine?

The influenza vaccine should be given to all children at risk of getting severe pneumonia from influenza infection. *In addition, the influenza vaccine should be given to all children and adults living in the home of someone at risk.* Diseases considered to put children at risk of severe pneumonia are summarized below:

1. Asthma. Children with asthma significant enough to require regular medical visits should be immunized.

2. Diabetes

3. Heart disease. Children with heart disease severe enough to cause congestive heart failure should be immunized.

4. Kidney disease

5. Sickle cell disease

6. Cystic fibrosis

7. Lung disease of prematurity (called bronchopulmonary dysplasia, or BPD)

8. AIDS or HIV infection

9. Cancer, lymphoma, or leukemia

10. Long-term aspirin therapy

Influenza Is Very Contagious

Up to 40 percent of people exposed to influenza will get sick.

If influenza is so dangerous, why not give the influenza vaccine to everybody?

Influenza virus regularly causes epidemics every one to three years, and proteins on the surface of the virus change as often as the epidemics. Because protection against influenza is caused by antibodies directed against these surface proteins, the influenza vaccine has to be updated yearly to include the new strains that are circulating that year.

In order for yearly mass immunization against influenza to effectively reduce the incidence of the virus in this country, nearly everyone would need to be vaccinated (including all adults). As our health care system is currently constructed, this would be difficult. Therefore, the vaccine is recommended only for those in high-risk groups.

Isn't there a new influenza vaccine given to children as nose drops?

There is an influenza vaccine that is given as a nasal spray. This vaccine is not yet licensed in the United States but has been tested in infants, children, and adults, with very promising results. The vaccine will probably be licensed in 1999. Because the vaccine is effective and easy to administer, it is possible that it would be recommended for *all* infants, children, and adults, and not just those at high risk of severe disease.

The Swine Flu

In 1976, public health officials discovered something alarming. In Fort Dix, New Jersey, there was an outbreak of influenza virus infection in military recruits caused by a strain (called "swine flu") very different from other circulating strains.

These kinds of strains often herald the beginning of influenza pandemics. Public health officials decided to immunize everyone in the country to try to prevent a nationwide outbreak.

Didn't the "swine flu" vaccine cause paralysis in some people?

The "swine flu" vaccine was administered in the United States in a mass immunization program in 1976 and was associated with a disease called Guillain-Barré syndrome in about 1 in 200,000 vaccine recipients. People with Guillain-Barré syndrome developed paralysis that began in the legs and spread to the arms and breathing muscles. Most people recovered without permanent damage.

Since 1976, about 15 to 18 million adults and children have been immunized with the influenza vaccine. If the influenza vaccine is a cause of Guillain-Barré syndrome (an association that is unproven), it does so at a rate of fewer than 1 case per 100,000 doses. The reasons for the association between "swine flu" vaccine and Guillain-Barré syndrome remain unclear.

INFLUENZA VACCINE: SUMMARY AND CONCLUSIONS

The influenza virus causes fever, muscle aches, headaches, and, in some children, severe pneumonia. Certain children are at very high risk of severe disease when they get infected. Because many people who would benefit from the vaccine don't get vaccinated (including children with asthma and their families), the influenza vaccine is probably the most underused in all of medicine.

CHAPTER 17

PNEUMOCOCCUS ("THE PNEUMONIA VACCINE")

Benjamin is 5 years old. Over the past three years he has been admitted to the hospital twice with pneumonia. His mother is frustrated by these admissions and asks the doctor about preventing this disease.

Is there a vaccine that can prevent pneumonia in children?

Pneumococcus is a bacterium that is now the most common cause of pneumonia, meningitis (inflammation of the lining of the brain), and sepsis (bloodstream infection causing shock) in young children. Every year, thousands of previously healthy children die or are permanently damaged by the diseases caused by this bacterium.

Given the impact of this infection, one would imagine that the pneumococcal vaccine would be part of a child's routine immunization series. Unfortunately, this is not the case. The problem with the current pneumococcal vaccine is that it doesn't work well in young children.

Since most severe pneumococcal infections occur in children under 2 years of age, the vaccine has limited usefulness.

The current vaccine is recommended only for those children over 2 years of age at high risk for getting severe pneumococcal infections. In this chapter we will talk about who should get the pneumococcal vaccine, why the vaccine doesn't work in the young children who need it, and prospects for a better vaccine.

Recommendations by the American Academy of Pediatrics

The pneumococcal vaccine is recommended for children older than 2 years of age at high risk of getting severe pneumococcal disease (see below).

The vaccine is given as a single shot. In children under 10 years of age, the vaccine should be given every three to five years.

What Is Pneumococcus?

Pneumococcus is a bacterium (*Streptococcus pneumoniae*) which is now the most common cause of pneumonia, meningitis, sepsis, ear infections, and sinusitis in children under 2 years of age.

Every year in the United States, pneumococcus causes about 50,000 cases of pneumonia, 5,000 cases of meningitis, and 30,000 cases of sepsis. Most of the cases in children occur in those younger than 2 years old. In addition, about 80 percent of children will have at least one episode of ear infection caused by pneumococcus by the time they are 3 years old.

Every year, thousands of children either die or are left permanently damaged from the diseases caused by this bacterium.

Pneumococcus Is Number One

Up until 1990, the bacterium Hib (*Haemophilus influenzae* type b) was the number-one cause of sepsis and meningitis in

continues

children younger than 2 years of age. In 1990, the Hib vaccine was released. Since then, the pneumococcus has become the most common cause of these diseases.

What Is the Pneumococcal Vaccine?

Pneumococcus is very similar to Hib. Both are bacteria coated with a sugar called polysaccharide. Protection against pneumococcus is caused by antibodies directed against this sugar. Unfortunately, infants and children younger than 2 years of age can't make antibodies to this sugar.

Researchers found that if you joined the sugar to a harmless protein (producing a so-called conjugate vaccine), children did develop immunity to the sugar. The Hib vaccine is made by joining the sugar to a protein. Unfortunately, this hasn't been easy to do with pneumococcus. Therefore, the current pneumococcal vaccine consists of only the sugar (the unconjugated vaccine).

Why was it easy to make a Hib vaccine but hard to make a pneumococcal vaccine? Whereas there is only one type of Hib, there are 90 types of pneumococcus—23 of which are in the vaccine. These 23 types cause about 90 percent of disease. It has been technically difficult to join all of the important pneumococcal types to proteins and put them into one vaccine.

Antibiotics Didn't Solve the Pneumococcus Problem

In the 1940s, antibiotics were developed and hailed as the final answer to the diseases caused by pneumococcus.

However, by 1960, tens of thousands of people were still dying every year from pneumococcus. Antibiotics didn't always work, because diseases such as sepsis and meningitis are sometimes rapid and overwhelming. In addition, some strains of pneumococcus have become very resistant to antibiotics. These observations have renewed interest in developing a pneumococcal vaccine.

Is the pneumococcal vaccine safe?

The pneumococcal vaccine occasionally causes pain or soreness where the shot was given. In addition, fewer than 1 percent of those immunized will develop low-grade fever and muscle aches.

Who should get the pneumococcal vaccine?

The pneumococcal vaccine should be given to children over 2 years of age who are at high risk of getting severe pneumococcal infections. This includes children with the following problems:

1. Sickle cell disease

2. Absence of a spleen. This includes children who have had their spleen removed after trauma.

3. Long-standing kidney disease

4. Diseases requiring treatment that weakens the immune system, such as cancer, leukemia, and lymphoma

5. HIV infection or AIDS

Some Children Are at Very High Risk of Pneumococcal Disease

Younger children without spleens are 13 times more likely to get severe pneumococcal infections than other children: for the HIV-infected child, the risk is 100 times greater, and for the preschool-age child with sickle cell disease the risk is 600 times greater.

If diseases caused by pneumococcus are so bad, why not give the vaccine to all children?

The pneumococcus bacterium kills about 40,000 people every year, many of them children younger than 2 years old.

Unfortunately, the current pneumococcal vaccine (or unconjugated vaccine) is ineffective in children under 2 years. Children in this age group simply do not have very good immune responses to the sugars, or polysaccharides, that coat pneumococcus. Even after a natural infection with pneumococcus, these children don't develop strong antibody responses.

Until researchers are successful at linking the many types of pneumococcal polysaccharides to proteins (to produce conjugated vaccines) for use in a single shot, children under 2 will continue to die from diseases caused by this bacterium.

When can we expect a better vaccine?

The long-awaited pneumococcal vaccine containing pneumococcal sugars joined to proteins will probably be available for use in children under 2 years of age by the year 2002.

PNEUMOCOCCAL VACCINE: SUMMARY AND CONCLUSIONS

The bacterium called pneumococcus causes pneumonia, meningitis, sepsis, ear infections, and sinusitis in children. Every year thousands of children die or are permanently disabled by infections caused by this bacterium. In addition, pneumococcus is becoming progressively more resistant to antibiotics. Unfortunately, the current pneumococcal vaccine doesn't work very well in younger children and therefore is recommended only for those over 2 years of age at particularly high risk of severe disease. A better vaccine should be available soon.

CHAPTER 18

MENINGOCOCCUS ("THE SEPSIS/ MENINGITIS VACCINE")

Amy is 14 years old. One day after school, she tells her mother that one of her classmates was in the hospital with meningitis. Two days later, Amy's mother discovers that the classmate had died of the disease.

Is Amy at risk of having caught meningitis from her classmate?

Are there vaccines that could prevent Amy from getting meningitis?

There is no infectious disease more terrifying to parents than the one caused by meningococcus.

A healthy child can progress from a mild rash and fever to shock, coma, and death within 12 hours. When meningococcus enters a child care center or school, the panic that spreads through a community is unlike that caused by any other illness.

Like pneumococcus and Hib, meningococcus usually infects children under 4 years of age. Unfortunately, as with pneumococcus, an effective vaccine for meningococcus has been difficult to develop for young children. Therefore, the meningococcal vaccine is used only for children older than 2 years of age at particularly high risk of infection.

In this chapter we will discuss who should get the meningococcal vaccine, whether the vaccine should be used during community outbreaks of infection, and the prospects for a better vaccine.

Recommendation by the American Academy of Pediatrics

The meningococcal vaccine is recommended for children older than 2 years of age at high risk for getting severe meningococcal disease (see below).

The vaccine is given as a single shot.

WHAT IS MENINGOCOCCUS?

Meningococcus is a bacterium (*Neisseria meningitidis*) that is a common cause of sepsis, a bloodstream infection causing low blood pressure and shock, and meningitis, infection of the lining of the brain, in children under 4 years of age. Every year in the United States, meningococcus causes about 3,000 cases of sepsis and meningitis.

The sepsis caused by meningococcus is often rapid and overwhelming. Healthy children can progress from a mild rash and fever to shock, coma, and death within 12 hours. Despite a quick medical response and appropriate therapy, as many as 30 percent of children with sepsis will die from the infection.

Children with meningitis caused by meningococcus often have symptoms similar to those with Hib: high fever, headache, drowsiness, and a stiff neck. About 1 in 20 children with meningococcal meningitis will die, and many of those who survive will be left with brain damage.

Epidemics of Meningococcus Happen Every Year

Every year in the United States, epidemics of sepsis and meningitis caused by meningococcus occur in child care centers and schools.

WHAT IS THE MENINGOCOCCAL VACCINE?

Meningococcus is similar to both pneumococcus and Hib. All three bacteria are coated with polysaccharide, and protection against disease is caused by antibodies directed against this sugar. Unfortunately, infants and children under 2 years of age can't develop immunity to this sugar.

Researchers found that if you joined sugars to harmless proteins, producing conjugate vaccines, children would make antibodies to the sugars. Unfortunately, the current unconjugated meningococcal vaccine consists only of the sugar.

Why was it easier to develop a Hib vaccine (meaning to conjugate the Hib sugar to a protein) than to make a meningococcal vaccine? Hib is different from meningococcus in that there is only one type of Hib that causes disease in children (Hib type b), whereas there are at least five different types of meningococcus (types A, B, C, Y, and W-135). In addition, it is very hard for either children or adults to produce antibodies to one meningococcal type—type B—the type that causes about half of the meningococcus outbreaks.

Therefore, the current meningococcal vaccine is unconjugated and contains only types A, C, Y, and W-135.

Is the meningococcal vaccine safe?

Yes. There are no serious side effects from the vaccine. However, the meningococcal vaccine does cause pain or soreness where the shot was given in about 4 percent of children.

Who should get the meningococcal vaccine?

The meningococcal vaccine should be given to children over 2 years of age who are at high risk of getting meningococcal infection. This includes children with the following very unusual problems or situations:

1. Absence of a spleen, as with children who have had their spleens removed following trauma.

2. Lack of a specific group of serum proteins (called complement proteins) that help the body fight infection.

3. Travel to sub-Saharan Africa during the dry season (December through June).

If meningococcal diseases are so bad, why not give the vaccine to all children?

The meningococcal vaccine has been hard to develop. To make a successful vaccine, researchers have tried to overcome two obstacles. First, they have to tried to devise a way to link all five types of meningococcus to proteins and put them in a single conjugate vaccine. This will probably happen by 2002.

The second and more difficult task is to find a way to get both children and adults to successfully respond to type B, the type that causes about half of all meningococcal disease. Meningococcus type B shares a substance called neuraminic acid that is identical to one on the surface of some fetal nervous system cells. Therefore, girls or women vaccinated against meningococcus type B (a type *not* included in the current vaccine) may inadvertently make antibodies directed against their future unborn child. This could have disastrous effects and may forever preclude the development of a vaccine that uses the sugar of meningococcus type B.

Until these significant problems in vaccine development are solved, younger children will continue to die from sepsis and meningitis caused by this bacterium.

There were recently two children in my son's school who had meningitis. The public health officer said that these children were infected with meningococcus. What should I do?

There are two things to do if your child is exposed to children in school who have meningitis caused by meningococcus.

First, an antibiotic (rifampin or ciprofloxacin) is recommended only for those children who either live in the home of an infected person or attend the same child care center or nursery school. *In elementary school or high school, one is considered to be exposed if the contact is intimate (meaning kissing or sharing food or beverages). Otherwise, children in school, church, or community center settings do not need antibiotics.*

Second, if an outbreak of meningitis in a school is caused by a type of meningococcus that is contained in the vaccine (type A, C, Y, or W-135), the vaccine may help protect children from getting infected. Therefore, parents should try to find out what type of bacteria is causing the outbreak of sepsis or meningitis in the child's school or day care center and follow the recommendations of local public health authorities.

If a child in school has meningitis caused by pneumococcus, neither antibiotics nor vaccines are recommended, because the risk of a spread to other children is so low.

MENINGOCOCCAL VACCINE: SUMMARY AND CONCLUSIONS

Every year in the United States, meningococcus causes thousands of cases of sepsis and meningitis in children under 4 years of age. Many of these children die or are left permanently disabled by these infections. Unfortunately, the current meningococcal vaccine is not very effective in preventing disease in younger children. Therefore, the vaccine is recommended only for those at particularly high risk of disease. The meningococcal vaccine may be of benefit in community outbreaks of infection.

CHAPTER 1 9

TUBERCULOSIS

Christopher is 6 years old. Christopher's mother learns one day that his 72-year-old uncle was recently diagnosed with tuberculosis. The uncle had been at a Christmas party at the house about three weeks ago.

What should Christopher's mother do? Is there a vaccine to prevent tuberculosis?

Recently there has been a resurgence of tuberculosis in this country. Although between 1950 and 1984 the incidence of the disease steadily declined, between 1985 and 1991 there were about 40,000 more cases than would have been predicted. The single most important reason for the increase in tuberculosis is the introduction of the AIDS virus into the United States. People with AIDS are at high risk of developing tuberculosis and spreading it to others.

Because the number of people with tuberculosis is increasing, and children are at increased risk of catching the disease, the Centers for Disease Control and Prevention recently reconsidered its policy on the tuberculosis vaccine. The results of that decision are described below.

Recommendation by the American Academy of Pediatrics

The tuberculosis vaccine is recommended only for children who live in very unusual situations. Children are recommended to receive the vaccine if they are in the same household as someone actively infected with tuberculosis who either (1) cannot take the antibiotics that treat tuberculosis or (2) is infected with a strain of bacteria that is very resistant to antibiotics. This situation currently applies to a very small number of children in this country.

WHAT IS TUBERCULOSIS?

Tuberculosis is a disease caused by a bacterium called *Mycobacterium tuberculosis*. This bacterium can infect every organ of the body, but most prominently infects the lungs.

People with tuberculosis infection of the lungs usually have a persistent, unrelenting cough. Occasionally the sputum brought up by the cough is streaked with blood. The patient also can develop sweating at night, loss of weight, and a progressive decrease in physical activity. If left untreated, the disease is often fatal (in the old days tuberculosis was called "consumption").

Children under 5 years of age will occasionally get a very severe form of tuberculosis associated with meningitis or a rapid, overwhelming, often fatal form of infection called miliary tuberculosis.

Many people become infected with tuberculosis without knowing it. They don't develop any symptoms of tuberculosis when they are first infected. However, as they get older, the bacteria can reawaken, or reactivate, and cause severe lung disease. The way to tell whether someone is infected is to do a skin test called PPD. Children living in or around an area where tuberculosis is present are usually tested two or three times by 5 years of age to see if they have been exposed to tuberculosis.

The Impact of Tuberculosis

Tuberculosis kills more people in the world than any other infection. It currently infects 1.7 billion people worldwide, about one-third of the world's population.

WHAT IS THE TUBERCULOSIS VACCINE?

Many parents are surprised to hear that there is a tuberculosis vaccine.

The tuberculosis vaccine is called BCG, which stands for Bacillus of Calmette and Guérin. It has been given to about 4 billion people. Since the 1960s, the only countries that have *not* routinely used the BCG vaccine are the United States and The Netherlands.

The BCG vaccine is made from a bacterium (called *Mycobacterium bovis*) that was originally isolated from cows by two French scientists, Calmette and Guérin, in 1908. The researchers reasoned that the cow tuberculosis bacterium was similar enough to the human tuberculosis bacterium that immunization with one would protect against disease caused by the other. They weakened this bovine tuberculosis strain by continually growing it in a nutrient broth for a period of 13 years.

In 1921, the vaccine was first used in humans. For the most part, the vaccine is not effective in preventing adolescents and adults from getting the lung disease caused by tuberculosis. However, it is effective about 80 percent of the time in preventing young children from getting the severe form of tuberculosis (meaning tuberculous meningitis or rapid, overwhelming tuberculosis infection).

Is the tuberculosis vaccine safe?

The tuberculosis vaccine is safe. About three out of every 10,000 children less than one year of age will develop a painful swelling of the glands under the arm that was injected with the vaccine. This swelling can last as long as three months.

How do you catch tuberculosis?

Tuberculosis can be very contagious. The disease is spread by tiny droplets produced by coughing, sneezing, or even talking. Up to 3,000 infectious droplets can be made after one cough, one sneeze, or talking for about five minutes.

Two outbreaks of tuberculosis in closed environments show just how contagious the disease can be. One person on the submarine *Byrd* infected 45 percent of the entire crew. Another, an elderly man in a nursing home, infected about 80 percent of the residents living in the same wing.

Who should get the tuberculosis vaccine?

The United States is trying to stop the spread of tuberculosis by treating with antibiotics those people who have disease of the lungs or who are silently infected with the bacteria. The hope is that vigorous identification of these infections and treatment with appropriate antibiotics will prevent the spread of tuberculosis. Because the vaccine is not effective in preventing infections in the lungs of adolescents and adults, BCG vaccine is not routinely used in the United States.

The vaccine is recommended only for children living in very unusual situations. Children are recommended to receive the vaccine if they are in the same household as someone who is actively infected with tuberculosis and either (1) cannot take the antibiotics that treat tuberculosis or (2) is infected with a strain of bacteria that is very resistant to antibiotics. This situation currently applies to only a very small number of children in this country.

What are we doing about tuberculosis in this country?

The United States uses two approaches to eliminate tuberculosis.

First, it seeks to eliminate the possibilities for spreading the disease by identifying people who are actively infected with tuberculosis and treating them with appropriate antibiotics. Although people who have severe tuberculosis infection of the lungs are very contagious, treatment with antibiotics (such as isoniazid, or INH, rifampin, ethambutal, and pyrazinamide) stops the shedding of bacteria within two weeks.

Second, it tries identify people who are silently infected with the tuberculosis bacterium and treat them with antibiotics. People who are silently infected have a positive skin test (PPD) but no symptoms.

Treating them with antibiotics such as INH makes it much less likely that the bacteria will reactivate and later cause disease of the lungs or other organs.

TUBERCULOSIS VACCINE: SUMMARY AND CONCLUSIONS

The tuberculosis vaccine is not very good at preventing infection of the lungs in teenagers and adults. Therefore, it is not routinely used in this country. However, because of the resurgence of tuberculosis in the United States, there are certain unusual situations in which the vaccine is now recommended. It is recommended for children who live in the same household as someone who has tuberculosis infection of the lungs if the infected person either can't take antibiotics or is infected with a strain of tuberculosis that is very resistant to antibiotics.

PART FOUR

VACCINES FOR CHILDREN WHO TRAVEL TO FAR-OFF LANDS

CHAPTER 20

SOURCES OF INFORMATION ABOUT VACCINES FOR TRAVELERS

In August of 1996, a Tennessee man came back from a fishing trip in South America and died of yellow fever. He was the first person to die of this disease in the United States in over 70 years. Although he knew that the yellow fever vaccine was recommended for travel to the Amazon Basin, he had chosen not to get it.

Traveling to other countries occasionally exposes one to microorganisms that are rarely, if ever, encountered in the United States. Many of these microorganisms are potentially deadly. Unfortunately, many travelers don't know how to find out about the diseases that are prevalent in different countries or about the vaccines available to prevent them. It is especially difficult to determine which vaccines can be safely taken by young children. Although travel agents and airlines are willing to inform traveler's about vaccines *required* for travel, rarely do they inform travelers about those that are *recommended* for travel.

So how can you get this information?

First, there are many travel clinics in this country that provide information about both infectious diseases in different parts of the world and the vaccines that prevent them. One can usually find out about the availability of these clinics from travel agents, doctors, or medical centers.

Second, a book published by the Centers for Disease Control and Prevention (CDC) called *Health Information for International Travel 1996–97* is available for sale from the Superintendent of Documents, Government Printing Office, Washington, DC 20402; (202) 512-1800. Unfortunately, patterns of diseases, especially in developing countries, can change fairly rapidly, and information in books can lose relevance.

Third, the CDC maintains a Web site that constantly updates information on vaccines both recommended and required for travel (http://www.cdc.gov).

Finally, the CDC has an updated voice information service at (404) 332-4559.

Many people who travel don't understand the difference between vaccines that are "required" and those that are "recommended." Most people believe that a vaccine is required to prevent disease from a likely exposure, and that a vaccine is recommended to prevent disease from an unlikely exposure. This interpretation is almost the exact opposite of the truth.

Vaccines are required because a country does not want its own citizens exposed to a particular disease. The requirement is an attempt to limit the importation of that disease into the country. On the other hand, vaccines are recommended because a disease is prevalent in a country and *visitors'* risk of exposure is high. To put it another way, vaccines are required to protect the people in the country you are visiting and vaccines are recommended to protect you, the visitor.

The chapters that follow contain detailed descriptions of the five vaccines that are available to prevent some of the diseases highly prevalent abroad: hepatitis A virus, cholera, typhoid, yellow fever, and Japanese encephalitis virus. It should also be noted that children *and* parents should be up to date on the ten vaccines that are universally recommended (measles, mumps, rubella, polio, diphtheria, pertussis, tetanus, hepatitis B, Hib, and varicella).

CHAPTER 21

HEPATITIS A

Fred is 5 years old. His parents are traveling to Jamaica and want to take Fred with them. They will be going to places in Jamaica with standard tourist accommodations and food.

Are there any vaccines that Fred should get before he leaves?

The hepatitis A virus is a common cause of hepatitis (inflammation of the liver). In the United States there are about 100,000 cases of hepatitis A every year. In developing countries in Asia, Africa, South America, Central America, the Caribbean, southern Europe, the Middle East (including Israel), the Mediterranean Basin, and Mexico the disease is common. Almost *all* adults living in developing countries have been infected at some time in their lives with the hepatitis A virus.

A vaccine to prevent the hepatitis A virus was licensed by the Food and Drug Administration in February of 1995. Because the virus is so prevalent in many areas of the world, all children traveling to developing countries (even if they plan to use standard tourist accommodations, itineraries, and food) should receive the hepatitis A vaccine.

> ## Recommendation by the American Academy of Pediatrics
>
> The hepatitis A virus vaccine is recommended for travel to *all* countries *except* Australia, Canada, Japan, New Zealand, Scandinavia, and countries in western Europe. Children traveling to all other countries (including Mexico and the Caribbean) should receive the vaccine.
>
> The vaccine is given to children at least 2 years of age in the form of two shots. The second shot is given 6 to 18 months after the first.

What Is Hepatitis A?

Hepatitis A is a virus that causes hepatitis, or inflammation of the liver. Children usually have fever, yellowing of the skin (jaundice), loss of appetite, nausea, and vomiting. The disease is rarely a cause of death or permanent liver damage in children.

What Is the Hepatitis A Vaccine?

The hepatitis A vaccine contains the whole virus that is killed by treatment with the chemical formaldehyde. Because the virus cannot replicate, it cannot cause hepatitis.

Is the hepatitis A vaccine safe?

Although it is relatively new, about 70,000 people have been given the hepatitis A vaccine without any serious side effects. About 10 percent of children will have pain where the shot was given.

In which countries can you catch hepatitis A?

Outbreaks of hepatitis A can occur in any country in the world. However, the disease is most prevalent in Asia, Africa, South America, Central America, the Middle East, the Mediterranean Basin, southern Europe, the Caribbean, and Mexico.

How can I avoid catching the hepatitis A virus?

In developing countries, the hepatitis A virus is transmitted by contaminated food or water. Travelers can best avoid catching the virus by avoiding uncooked shellfish, uncooked or peeled fruits or vegetables, beverages with ice, or water of unknown purity.

Unfortunately, many persons catch the hepatitis A virus while traveling to countries where the disease is prevalent despite standard tourist accommodations, itineraries, and foods. Therefore, the vaccine is recommended for *all* persons traveling to those countries.

Why Shellfish Contain the Hepatitis A Virus

In order to obtain adequate quantities of food, shellfish (such as oysters, mussels, clams, crabs, and lobsters) filter hundreds of quarts of water every day. Hepatitis A virus (present in the water) is concentrated in the shellfish.

Who should get the hepatitis A virus vaccine?

The hepatitis A virus vaccine is not required for international travel, but it is *recommended* for *all* children over 2 years of age who are traveling to countries where the disease is highly prevalent.

I am going to Mexico with my 5-year-old son, and we are leaving in one week. Do I have enough time to get my son vaccinated with the hepatitis A vaccine?

A period of at least four weeks is required for about 90 percent of children to become protected against disease after getting the vaccine. Therefore, parents should make every effort to give their children the vaccine at least four weeks before traveling. However, many children are probably protected against hepatitis A virus infection within two weeks of the first dose of vaccine. So it is still worth getting the hepatitis A vaccine even if you know you are traveling within two weeks.

To ensure protection against the hepatitis A virus for children whose travel is imminent (meaning within four weeks), it is also of value to inject immunoglobulin (antibodies directed against hepatitis A virus) at the same time that the vaccine is given. Unfortunately, the national supply of immunoglobulin is low. Because of this shortage, it is now more important than ever that parents plan to give their children the hepatitis A vaccine well before departure.

For long-term protection against hepatitis A virus infection (at least ten years), both shots are required.

I am traveling to Nassau in the Bahamas with my daughter, who is only 15 months old. Is she too young to get the hepatitis A vaccine?

The hepatitis A vaccine is not recommended for children under 2 years of age. Parents traveling to areas where the hepatitis A virus is prevalent (including the Bahamas) should have their doctor give a single shot of immunoglobulin, antibodies directed against hepatitis A virus, prior to travel. The immunoglobulin will protect the child for up to three months.

HEPATITIS A VACCINE: SUMMARY AND CONCLUSIONS

The hepatitis A virus is a common cause of hepatitis worldwide. Although the disease is rarely fatal, the symptoms can be quite disabling.

The hepatitis A virus is so prevalent worldwide that it is easier to list countries where you don't need the vaccine than those where you do need it. Children over 2 years of age traveling to *all* countries *except* Australia, Canada, Japan, New Zealand, Scandinavia, and countries in western Europe should receive the vaccine.

CHAPTER 22

CHOLERA

Kurt is 9 years old. Kurt's parents are planning to take him with them on their trip to India. They have read in newspapers that there are continually outbreaks of cholera in India.

Is there a cholera vaccine? If so, should Kurt get the vaccine?

Cholera is a cause of severe diarrhea and water loss, or dehydration, in India, Southeast Asia, Africa, the Middle East, southern Europe, the western Pacific Islands (Oceania), South America, and some parts of central Asia. Every year more than one million people are infected and about 100,000 die from cholera. Most of these cases occur in Asia and Africa.

Travelers using standard tourist accommodations to areas where cholera is prevalent are at virtually no risk of disease.

No country requires the cholera vaccine for entry.

Recommendation by the American Academy of Pediatrics

The cholera vaccine is not required for entry into any country, nor is it recommended for those who stay (in standard tourist accommodations) in areas where the disease is prevalent.

CHOLERA

WHAT IS CHOLERA?

Cholera is a bacterium (*Vibrio cholera*) that infects the intestines. Most people infected with cholera have no symptoms, but some (about 5 percent) have severe diarrhea. The diarrhea caused by cholera can be so severe that a person can go into shock within four hours of the beginning of illness.

A Death in Venice

For several years now Asiatic cholera had shown a heightened tendency to spread and migrate . . . in the middle of this May in Venice the frightful vibrions were found on one and the same day in the blackish wasted bodies of a cabin boy and a woman who sold greengroceries. The cases were kept secret. But within a week there were ten, twenty, thirty more, and in various sections . . . the food supply had been infected. . . . Cases of recovery were rare. Out of a hundred attacks, eighty were fatal, and in the most horrible manner. For the plague moved with utter savagery. . . .

From Thomas Mann's *Death in Venice*, 1930.

WHAT IS THE CHOLERA VACCINE?

The cholera vaccine is composed of whole cholera bacteria that have been inactivated, or killed, with a chemical. The vaccine is not highly effective (the vaccine protects against disease only about 50 percent of the time) and doesn't contain one of the types of bacteria that is currently circulating in India, Bangladesh, and parts of central Asia and eastern Europe. Because of this, all travelers who receive the vaccine should still be very careful to eat food that is properly cooked and drink only bottled water.

Is the cholera vaccine safe?

The cholera vaccine has a high rate of mild side effects. Vaccination often results in one to two days of pain, tenderness, and redness where the shot was given. These local reactions may also be accompanied by fever, headache, and fatigue. Serious reactions are extremely rare.

In which countries can you catch cholera?

Cholera continues to cause disease in India, Southeast Asia, Africa, the Middle East, southern Europe, the western Pacific Islands (Oceania), South America, and some states of the former Soviet Union (including Ukraine, Azerbaijan, and Armenia).

How can I avoid catching cholera?

Travelers using standard tourist accommodations are at virtually no risk of disease.

However, because the bacterium is spread in water and food (primarily shellfish), the best way to avoid cholera is to make sure that non-bottled water is boiled and that shellfish are adequately cooked.

Who should get the cholera vaccine?

The vaccine is not recommended for use by the World Health Organization, nor is it required for entry into any country. However, some local authorities continue to require cholera vaccination. In such cases, a single dose of the cholera vaccine is sufficient.

CHOLERA VACCINE: SUMMARY AND CONCLUSIONS

Cholera is a common cause of severe diarrhea and death in a number of developing countries. However, travelers using standard tourist accommodations are at virtually no risk of disease. Therefore, the vaccine is not recommended by the World Health Organization, nor is it required for entry by any country.

TYPHOID

Robert is 13 years old. His parents want to take Robert with them on their trip to Mexico. They have heard that typhoid fever is common in Mexico and wonder whether there is a vaccine to prevent it.

Typhoid is a disease caused by a bacterium, *Salmonella typhi*. The bacterium causes fever, stomach pain, rash, and in some cases shock and death (called typhoid fever). It is estimated that every year there are 33 million cases of typhoid fever and 500,000 deaths worldwide. The disease primarily occurs in Mexico and the developing countries of South America, South and East Asia, and Africa.

The typhoid vaccine is not required for international travel, but it is recommended to travelers (under certain circumstances) in areas where the disease is prevalent.

Recommendation by the American Academy of Pediatrics

The typhoid vaccine is not required for international travel. The vaccine is recommended for anyone traveling to areas of high

continues

151

risk who is *likely to travel to small towns and rural areas or is unlikely to live and eat in standard tourist accommodations.* In addition, the vaccine is recommended for anyone staying for more than six weeks in areas where typhoid is common.

There are three typhoid vaccines. Their use depends on the age of the child.

- *6 years old or older:* One capsule by mouth of the "Ty21a" vaccine given every other day, for a total of four capsules.

- *2 to 6 years of age:* One shot of the purified "polysaccharide" vaccine.

- *6 months to 2 years of age:* Two shots of the "inactivated" vaccine, given at least four weeks apart.

The typhoid vaccine is not recommended for infants under 6 months of age.

WHAT IS TYPHOID?

Typhoid is a disease caused by a bacterium. The bacterium initially infects the intestines and causes fever, stomach pain, rash, and occasionally shock and death.

"Typhoid Mary"

Mary Mallon ("Typhoid Mary") was infected with typhoid bacteria in the early 1900s while living in New York. Although Mary never had any symptoms, she was contagious to others.

Unfortunately, Mary was a cook who refused to give up her occupation even after many warnings by the health department. She contaminated the food of probably hundreds of people, at least three of whom died of typhoid.

Mary spent the last 15 years of her life quarantined in a New York City hospital and died in 1930.

What Is the Typhoid Vaccine?

There are three typhoid vaccines. The choice of vaccines depends upon the age of the child.

- The *oral* vaccine (Ty21a) is a weakened form of the live bacteria.

- The *polysaccharide* vaccine is made of the sugar that coats the bacteria in the same way that the pneumococcal and meningococcal vaccines are made.

- The *inactivated* vaccine is a killed preparation of whole bacteria. The bacteria are killed by treatment with a chemical (phenol) and heat.

All three vaccines are between 50 and 80 percent effective at preventing typhoid.

Is the typhoid vaccine safe?

Both the oral and the polysaccharide vaccines are associated with far fewer side effects than the inactivated vaccine. The inactivated vaccine causes fever, headache, and pain where the shot is given in about 25 percent of recipients. Very rarely the "inactivated" typhoid vaccine causes low blood pressure and shock.

In which countries can you catch typhoid?

Typhoid is a cause of disease and death primarily in Mexico and in developing countries in East and South Asia (including India and Pakistan), South America, and Africa.

How can I avoid catching typhoid?

Typhoid is a disease of humans only and is transmitted through the feces. In developing countries, where sewage systems are poor, the disease is transmitted in contaminated water or food. Travelers should drink only bottled water and avoid ice, unpeeled fruit, undercooked meat, shellfish, salads, or food from street vendors.

The risk of disease is small if travel is limited to tourist accommodations.

Who should get the typhoid vaccine?

Anyone traveling to the developing countries listed above who is likely to enter small towns and rural areas, is staying for more than six weeks, or is unlikely to live and eat in tourist accommodations.

TYPHOID VACCINE:
SUMMARY AND CONCLUSIONS

Typhoid is a bacterium that causes fever, stomach pain, rash, and occasionally shock and death. There are more than 33 million cases and 500,000 deaths each year in the world. The disease is prevalent in developing countries in Asia, South America, and Latin America.

The typhoid vaccines used today are safe and fairly effective. However, because careful travelers are at low risk of catching the disease, the vaccine is recommended only for those who are likely to be exposed to contaminated food or water, those staying for long periods of time, or those staying in rural areas or small towns.

CHAPTER 24

YELLOW FEVER

David is 3 years old. His parents are planning a trip to Peru and have heard from friends that you can catch yellow fever in South America. They are reassured that the yellow fever vaccine is not required for entry.

If the yellow fever vaccine is not required for entry to Peru, does this also mean that it wouldn't be useful?

Yellow fever is one of the main causes of hepatitis (inflammation of the liver) and hemorrhage (a bleeding disorder) in parts of Africa and South America. Every year throughout the world there are about 200,000 cases of yellow fever, causing as many as 40,000 deaths. There are a number of countries where the vaccine is either required or recommended for use prior to entry.

Recommendation by the American Academy of Pediatrics

The yellow fever vaccine is either required or recommended for travel to a number of countries in Africa and South America. It is given as a single shot to children over 9 months of age.

WHAT IS YELLOW FEVER?

Yellow fever is a virus that causes inflammation of the liver (hepatitis) as well as severe bleeding problems (hemorrhage). Children usually have fever, chills, muscle pains, headache, and a yellowing of the skin (jaundice). Up to 20 percent of patients with jaundice will die from the disease.

WHAT IS THE YELLOW FEVER VACCINE?

The yellow fever vaccine is made in eggs, using a live, weakened form of the virus.

Is the yellow fever vaccine safe?

Side effects from the yellow fever vaccine are rare. About 5 percent of children who receive the vaccine will develop muscle pains and low-grade fever. However, because the vaccine is made in eggs, children with egg allergies should not get the vaccine.

In which countries can you catch yellow fever?

Yellow fever is found primarily in Africa and South America. The countries that require a certificate of vaccination for entry from the United States include Benin, Burkina Faso, Cameroon, Central African Republic, Congo, Ivory Coast, French Guiana, Gabon, Ghana, Liberia, Mali, Mauritania, Niger, Rwanda, Senegal, São Tomé, Principe, and Togo.

Countries in South America where yellow fever is prevalent include Brazil, Bolivia, Peru, Equador, Colombia, Panama, Venezuela, Guyana, Suriname, and French Guiana.

How can I avoid catching yellow fever?

Yellow fever is transmitted to children and adults by the bite of a mosquito. The disease is rarely transmitted in urban areas.

Travelers can avoid mosquito bites by staying in air-conditioned or well-screened quarters and wearing long-sleeved shirts and long pants. Insect repellents containing DEET should be used only on exposed skin, and repellents containing permethrin should be applied to clothing.

Mosquitoes are most active at sunset and dusk. Therefore, parents should choose indoor or protected activities for their children during these times of the day.

Who should get the yellow fever vaccine?

The yellow fever vaccine is required by the countries listed above and recommended for travel outside of urban areas in countries where the disease is prevalent. A single dose of vaccine provides protection against yellow fever for at least ten years and possibly a lifetime. The vaccine should not be given to pregnant women.

Although the vaccine is recommended only for children over 9 years of age, children under 9 traveling to the countries listed above may benefit from it if maximal protection against mosquito bites cannot be assured. Infants under 4 months of age should not receive the vaccine in any case because of the increased risk of severe side effects (specifically, encephalitis, or inflammation of the brain).

YELLOW FEVER VACCINE: SUMMARY AND CONCLUSIONS

Every year throughout the world there are about 200,000 cases of yellow fever. The disease is primarily located in certain countries in Africa and South America. Although a certificate of yellow fever vaccination is required for entry into a number of countries, there are also many other countries where administration of the vaccine would be of benefit prior to travel.

JAPANESE ENCEPHALITIS VIRUS

George is 8 years old. His father is being transferred by his company to Japan. The family plans to live in Japan for two years before coming back to the United States.

Are there any vaccines specific for travel to the Far East from which George may benefit?

Japanese encephalitis virus (JEV) is an occasional cause of outbreaks of encephalitis, inflammation of the brain, primarily in the Far East. Every year there are about 50,000 cases of JEV in the world. Of the children infected with this virus, one in four will die, and half of those who survive will be left with permanent brain damage.

The JEV vaccine is not required for international travel, but it is recommended for travel to certain areas dependent upon the length of stay, specific regions visited, and activities planned during travel.

> ## Recommendations by the American Academy of Pediatrics
>
> The Japanese encephalitis vaccine is recommended for children traveling to areas where the virus is prevalent whose length of stay or specific regions of travel (specifically rural or farming areas) put them at high risk. The vaccine should be given to children at least one year of age as a series of three shots. The last two shots are given seven and 30 days after the first shot.

WHAT IS JEV?

JEV is a virus that causes inflammation of the brain (encephalitis). Afflicted children usually have fever, headache, neck stiffness, nausea, and vomiting. Some children (about 25 percent) will progress to coma and death. Of those who survive, about 50 percent will have seizures and permanent brain damage.

WHAT IS THE JEV VACCINE?

The JEV vaccine is a live, weakened virus originally isolated in 1935. The virus is grown in cells from mouse brains, and the vaccine is made by purifying the virus and killing it with formaldehyde.

Is the JEV vaccine safe?

About 20 percent of children given the JEV vaccine will have fever or pain where the shot is given. About 10 percent will have fever, headache, malaise, rash, chills, dizziness, muscle pain, nausea, vomiting, or abdominal pain. About 0.5 percent of vaccinees will have a severe allergic reaction to the JEV vaccine (hives, difficulty breathing).

Because the virus is grown in mouse brains, there has always been concern that the virus may cause side effects in the nervous system. However, this has not been the case.

In which countries can you catch JEV?

JEV is found primarily in Bangladesh, Brunei, Burma, Cambodia, Hong Kong, India, Indonesia, Japan, Korea, Laos, Malaysia, Nepal, the

People's Republic of China, Pakistan, the Philippines, Russia, Singapore, Sri Lanka, Taiwan, Thailand, and Vietnam.

How can I avoid catching JEV?

JEV is transmitted to children by the bite of a mosquito. The disease is usually transmitted in the summer and early fall (in temperate climates), when mosquitoes are most likely to feed. Mosquitoes usually feed at night, between dusk and dawn.

Travelers can avoid JEV by staying in screened or air-conditioned rooms at dusk and at night. If that is not possible, they should use mosquito netting over beds, as well as insect repellent and protective clothing.

Who should get the JEV vaccine?

The JEV vaccine is not required for international travel, but it is recommended in certain situations.

Travelers to countries listed above who are staying in urban areas or are staying for less than 30 days are at very low risk of catching JEV and are not recommended to receive the vaccine. On the other hand, travelers to those countries who will be (1) staying in rural or farm areas, (2) staying for more than 30 days, or (3) planning activities such as biking, camping, or other unprotected outdoor activities should consider having the vaccine.

Travelers should call either local travel clinics or the Centers for Disease Control and Prevention in Atlanta (404-332-4559) to determine in which seasons JEV would likely be prevalent in their destination.

JAPANESE ENCEPHALITIS VACCINE: SUMMARY AND CONCLUSIONS

Every year about 50,000 people in the world are infected with Japanese encephalitis virus. Many either die or are left with permanent brain damage from this infection. There are a number of countries in the Far East where the virus either circulates all the time or occurs in epidemics. For travelers to these countries, the vaccine is not required when travel will be confined to urban areas and will be for less than 30 days.

However, if travel will include rural areas or last for longer than one month, the Japanese encephalitis vaccine should be considered. The best way to make this decision is to call the Centers for Disease Control and Prevention at the number listed above and determine the months in which the virus is prevalent in your area of travel.

CHAPTER 26

THINGS TO THINK ABOUT WHEN TRAVELING WITH CHILDREN

FLYING AND JET LAG

During take-offs and landings, rapid changes in altitude may cause pressure and pain behind the eardrum. This can be prevented or lessened by giving the older child hard candy or chewing gum and the younger child a cup or bottle. The swallowing and chewing will equalize the pressure and prevent ear pain.

Crossing time zones and spending many hours in a plane can be a problem for even the most experienced adult traveler. Jet lag can cause tiredness, headaches, and irritability, which can lead to a crying, difficult-to-handle preschooler. However, medicines to make children sleepy during the plane ride are not recommended. In some children the medicines have the opposite effect, causing the child to be anxious, hyperactive, and unreasonable.

ALTITUDE (OR MOUNTAIN) SICKNESS

Up to one-third of persons who travel to high altitudes get symptoms of mountain sickness. The illness develops as the body adjusts to the lower oxygen levels in the air that occur at high altitudes. It may take a few hours to a couple of days to develop. Mountain sickness causes headache, poor appetite, dizziness, sleeplessness, and nausea. It is more common in young children than adults.

One of the medicines used to prevent or treat mild altitude or mountain sickness is called acetazolamide (Diamox®). This should be part of your travel medical kit if you plan to venture to altitudes of more than 10,000 feet (3050 meters). A bedtime dose is especially helpful for those who are having difficulty sleeping. Ask your doctor about the dose of acetazolamide and about whether this medicine would be right for your child.

FOOD, WATER, AND TRAVELER'S DIARRHEA

Even when care is taken in selecting food and drink, traveler's diarrhea is a common problem for most travelers. Children, especially preschoolers, are probably more likely to get it because of their mobility, natural curiosity, and hand-to-mouth behavior. Traveler's diarrhea is usually caused by a bacterium called enterotoxic *E. coli*.

The symptoms of traveler's diarrhea start with stomach cramps, followed by watery diarrhea. There may be fever, headaches, and tiredness. The diarrhea may occur many times a day and cause severe dehydration (water loss), especially in smaller children.

Fortunately, there are several simple rules to follow to avoid getting infected with the organisms that cause traveler's diarrhea. First, you should avoid the foods listed below:

"Boil It, Cook It, Peel It, or Forget It"

- Avoid foods that are raw or not thoroughly cooked, especially rare meats.

- Avoid fruits that cannot be peeled, such as apples, pears, and peaches.

- Avoid salads or uncooked vegetables.

- Avoid shellfish or raw, pickled, or undercooked seafood.

- Avoid food from street vendors.

Second, only bottled, purified, or carbonated water or other carbonated beverages should be used (with no ice). This includes water used for brushing teeth or taking medicines. If you are unable to purchase bottled or purified water, you need to purify the water yourself. This is done by adding five drops of tincture of iodine (2 percent) to one quart (or one liter) of water and letting the water stand for 30 minutes. The water is then safe to use. If the water is cloudy or cold, you should add ten drops. Tincture of iodine (2 percent) can be purchased from any drugstore.

If your child gets traveler's diarrhea, trimethoprim-sulfamethoxazole (Bactrim™, Septra®), which treats the most common cause of traveler's diarrhea, should be started. Medicines such as atropine (Lomotil®), loperamide (Imodium®), and diphenoxylate (Lomotil®), which decrease the number of bowel movements but do nothing to kill the bacteria, are not recommended for young children.

When your child becomes ill, the most important thing to avoid is dehydration. This can be avoided by giving your child plenty of fluids to drink. In most countries, oral rehydration liquids (such as Pedialyte®) are sold in drugstores or markets; these should be used for infants under 6 months of age. For older children, fluids such as carbonated caffeine-free beverages or canned fruit juices or soups can be used. Seek medical advice if you are concerned that the child is becoming less active, if diarrhea is more frequent than eight to ten watery stools a day, if the mouth and tongue become dry, if the child's frequency of urination significantly decreases, or if the diarrhea contains blood or mucus.

HEAT ILLNESS AND SUNSTROKE

Children are more likely to get heat illness than adults because they don't sweat as quickly in hot, humid climates. Travel to tropical or sub-tropical climates may result in cramping (heat cramps) or tiredness and dehydration (heat exhaustion).

Heat illnesses can be prevented by wearing loose-fitting cotton clothing, drinking plenty of fluids, and spending as much time as possible in the shade. Sunscreen (PABA-free, SPF 15 or higher) and avoidance of long periods of time in direct sunlight are important, especially for babies and toddlers.

When thirst, fatigue, and, in more severe cases, confusion occurs (symptoms of sunstroke), it is vital to move the child into a cool or shaded environment. Plenty of fluids should be given. Wetting the child's skin and hair with water and fanning to promote evaporation is helpful. If vomiting occurs and fluids can't be given, seek medical care.

BITES AND STINGS

Many unusual illnesses are transmitted by flying insects. The most common one is malaria, which is spread by the bite of mosquitoes (see next section). Travel to rural areas increases the chance of exposure to these diseases, but even in larger cities care should be taken. Insect repellents for skin and clothing and mosquito netting while sleeping will be necessary for some travelers, especially those traveling to some areas of Africa, Central and South America, and other tropical regions. Because mosquitoes most commonly bite between dusk and dawn, outdoor activity during those times should be avoided.

To reduce the number of mosquito bites, travelers should remain in well-screened areas, use mosquito netting while sleeping, and wear long pants and long-sleeved shirts when possible. In addition, insect repellents can be used on all exposed skin. The most effective repellents are those that contain the chemical called DEET. Adults and teenagers should use repellents with 30 to 35 percent DEET but not more concentrated repellents because of side effects (such as skin rashes). The DEET concentration for children in repellents should be even less, not more than 6 to 10 percent. The label lists the percentage of DEET contained in the product. "Skedaddle® Insect Protection for Children" (10 percent DEET), made by Little Point Corporation (Cambridge, Massachusetts), is one such product.

Greater degrees of protection against ticks, mosquitoes, and other insects is possible if clothes are sprayed or soaked in a powerful repellent called permethrin and then dried. Tents and mosquito netting can also be sprayed. An example of this product is Pemanone Tick Repellent (in a pressurized spray can) by Coulston International Corporation (Easton, Pennsylvania).

Unfortunately, spiders and hymenoptera (bees, wasps, hornets, and yellow jackets) are not repelled by DEET. If stung, check to see if the stinger is in place. If so, remove it while careful not to squeeze the venom sacs at the end of the stinger. Then give an antihistamine, such as Benadryl®, and apply cool compresses to the affected area. If the child has had severe reactions to stings in the past, an easy-to-carry, self-injecting epinephrine (EpiPen®) for emergency use should be prescribed by your doctor.

A summary of some of the unusual and exotic diseases spread by biting insects is shown below:

Exotic Diseases Caused by Bites and Stings

Disease	Insect	Location
Filariasis	Mosquitoes	Central & South America, Asia, Africa, Indian Subcontinent
Leishmaniasis	Sand flies	Central & South America, Africa, Europe, Indian Subcontinent
Onchocerciasis (River blindness)	Black flies	South America, Africa

Disease	Insect	Location
American Trypanosomiasis (Chagas disease)	Kissing bugs	South and Central America
African Trypanosomiasis (sleeping sickness)	Tsetse flies	West, Central, and East Africa
Barthonellosis (Oroya Fever)	Sand flies	South America
Yellow Fever	Mosquitoes	Tropical South America, Africa
Plague	Fleas	Asia, South America, Western North America
Relapsing Fever	Lice, Ticks	South America, Africa, Asia, Western North America
Chikungunya Fever	Mosquitoes	Africa, Southeast Asia, Indian subcontinent
Oropouche Virus Fever	Gnats	Brazil, Panama, Trinidad
Ross River Virus	Mosquitoes	Australia, South Pacific Islands
Congo-Crimean Tick Hemorrhagic Fever	Ticks	Eastern Europe, Central Asia, Indian subcontinent, Africa
Rift Valley Fever	Mosquitoes	Africa

PREVENTING MALARIA

Malaria is caused by a parasite that is transmitted from one person to another by the bite of an infected mosquito. Because mosquitoes bite from dusk to dawn, repellent and protection with mosquito netting at night is necessary. Malaria, and the mosquito that carries the disease, are present in all tropical and subtropical countries.

Malaria can cause fever, headaches, muscle aches, and tiredness (symptoms similar to those of flu). In rare instances, children can die from a severe malaria infection. Fortunately, malaria can be prevented by anti-malarial drugs such as chloroquine, mefloquine, and doxycycline. The medicine taken depends on the area of travel and the child's weight and age. All children (even infants) traveling to areas with malaria should take anti-malarial drugs.

THE YOUNG TRAVELER'S MEDICAL KIT

Below are some of the over-the-counter items that should be included in your visit to foreign countries.

The Young Traveler's Medical Kit		
Item	*Recommended product*	*For treatment of*
Analgesics	acetaminophen (Tylenol®, Tempra®, Panadol®)	Pain and fever
Antibiotics	trimethoprim-sulfa (Bactrim™, Septra®)	Traveler's diarrhea
Antihistamines	diphenhydramine (Benadryl®)	Bites and stings
	chloroquine, mefloquine, or doxycycline	Malaria
Antipyretics	ibuprofen (Motrin®, Advil®)	Pain and fever
Creams	hydrocortisone cream 1%	Bites and stings
First-aid supplies	bandages, tape, scissors, topical antibiotic creams	
	acetazolamide (Diamox®)	Prevention or treatment of mild "mountain sickness"
Insect repellents	DEET (10% concentration)	
Rehydration fluids	Pedialyte®	Diarrhea in infants
Sunscreen	PABA-free, SPF 15 or higher	Sun protection
Water purifier	Tincture of iodine 2%	

PART FIVE

VACCINES FOR CHILDREN IN THE FUTURE

CHAPTER 27

COMBINATION VACCINES

Trent is 2 months old. His mother takes him to the pediatrician and finds out that he needs four vaccines, all of which are given as shots (DTaP, Hib, Hep B, and IPV). She asks the doctor whether there is some way he can get these vaccines without getting so many shots.

There are ten vaccines that are recommended for routine use in all children. Of those ten vaccines, six are given in combination. The diphtheria, tetanus, and pertussis vaccines are combined to make DTaP; and the measles, mumps, and rubella vaccines are combined to make MMR. However, the recent addition of new vaccines such as Hib, varicella, hepatitis B, and the inactivated polio vaccine (IPV) have dramatically increased the number of shots that a child receives in the first year of life. It is now possible for a child to receive as many as four shots in a single visit (DTaP, IPV, Hib, and hepatitis B). This can be distressing to both the child and the parent.

Sometimes parents will ask their doctors whether they can draw up each of the different vaccines into a single syringe and give it to their child as a single shot. Unfortunately, it's not that easy. Sometimes either the stabilizer or buffer for one vaccine (and even the vaccine itself) will interfere with the capacity of another vaccine to induce immunity. Interestingly, this can also work in the other direction. For example, the "old" pertussis vaccine (used in the vaccine called DTP) probably enhanced the immune response to the diphtheria and tetanus components of the vaccine.

The good news is that help is on the way. Several companies are now working together to combine vaccines. The following combinations are either recently licensed or in progress:

- Probably the most useful combination vaccine (one that includes a combination of DTaP, Hib, hepatitis B, and IPV) will be available by 2000.

- A combination of hepatitis B and Hib was licensed in October of 1996 and became available in early 1997.

- A combination of DTaP and hepatitis B will probably be available in 1998.

- A combination of DTaP and Hib is now available for use as the fourth dose (given at about 15 months of age) and may be available for all doses by 1998.

- A combination of DTaP and IPV is now available in Europe and should be available in the United States in 1999.

- A combination of DTaP, IPV, and Hib may be available in the United States by 1999.

- A combination of DTaP, IPV, and Hep B should be available by 1999.

- A combination of Hib, Hep B, and IPV should also be available by 2001.

- A combination of measles, mumps, rubella, and varicella is currently being tested in clinical trials and could be available by 2002.

Use of these combination vaccines will clearly lessen the number of shots required in the first year.

CHAPTER 28

ROTAVIRUS ("THE DIARRHEA VACCINE")

Will is 14 months old. One day in February, he comes down with a high fever, diarrhea, and vomiting. Despite all her efforts, Will's mother can't get him to hold down even sips of juice. When the doctor examines Will, he notes that the boy's mouth and lips are dry and that when he cries there are no tears. Will's mother tells the doctor that Will hasn't wet his diaper for a day. The doctor says that Will is so dehydrated that he needs to come into the hospital to get fluids intravenously (IV).

Is there anything that can be done to prevent this from happening to other children?

Most parents are aware of the fact that during the winter months their young children may have a bout with diarrhea. What many parents don't know is that the most common cause of fever, vomiting, and diarrhea in children under 3 years of age has a name: rotavirus.

Every winter in the United States, rotavirus will infect about 2 million infants and young children. Because the virus causes both fever and vomiting (in addition to the diarrhea), it is often difficult to give children all the fluids they need. The result is that about 80,000 children will be admitted to the hospital every year in the United States with dehydration (water loss) caused by rotavirus. *That means that 1 out of every 50 children born in this country will be hospitalized with rotavirus infection.*

A new vaccine to prevent severe rotavirus disease may be available for use in infants by 1998.

WHAT IS ROTAVIRUS?

Rotavirus is a virus that infects the intestines. The infection causes fever, vomiting, and diarrhea lasting for about one week. Those most severely infected are between 6 months and 2 years of age.

Rotavirus infections are so common that *every* child in this country will be infected at least once by 3 years of age. Many children are infected two or three times within the first few years of life.

WHAT IS THE ROTAVIRUS VACCINE?

The strategy used to make the rotavirus vaccine is different from that for any other vaccine. The vaccine is a combination of strains of rotavirus that cause disease in children and strains that infect animals (specifically calves or monkeys).

Practically every mammal on earth is infected by its own unique rotavirus strains. So rotavirus not only infects children, it also infects the young of many other species. However, the rotavirus that infects one species isn't very efficient at infecting the young of another. For example, although cow (or bovine) rotavirus can cause severe diarrhea in calves, it doesn't cause diarrhea in children.

The rotavirus vaccine is made by combining either a bovine rotavirus or a monkey rotavirus with a human rotavirus (called a combination or reassortant virus). The human-bovine or human-monkey reassortant viruses have two important features. The human part of the reassortant viruses causes immunity that protects children against severe disease. The bovine or monkey part of the reassortant virus weakens the virus so that children don't get sick from the vaccine.

Is the rotavirus vaccine safe?

The rotavirus vaccine is safe. Fewer than 5 percent of infants given the vaccine may develop low-grade fever after the first dose.

Why should we prevent a disease as mild as diarrhea?

The disease caused by rotavirus is usually not mild.

The reason that rotavirus infections are so severe is that most infected children have both vomiting and fever in addition to the diarrhea. This means that not only do children lose fluids because of high fevers and diarrhea, but it is also difficult to replace the fluids lost because of the vomiting. Sometimes rotavirus infections are so severe that children become dehydrated within one day of the beginning of symptoms.

Who will get the rotavirus vaccine?

The rotavirus vaccine will probably be given to children at 2, 4, 6, and 15 to 18 months of age. It will be given as drops in the mouth.

When will I be able to give a rotavirus vaccine to my children?

The rotavirus vaccine has been tested in thousands of children between 2 months and 1 year of age and has been shown to be effective at preventing moderate-to-severe rotavirus disease. It may be available for use in all children as early as 1998.

Will the rotavirus vaccine prevent my child from getting diarrhea?

The rotavirus vaccine will prevent severe cases of rotavirus disease but not all cases of the disease. Some children who get the rotavirus vaccine may still get a mild case of diarrhea. However, because the vaccine eliminates the severe vomiting and high fevers caused by the virus, hospital admissions, doctors' visits, and emergency room visits for rotavirus will be reduced.

It should be noted that the rotavirus vaccine won't prevent diarrhea caused by other viruses and bacteria. However, because rotaviruses are the most important cause of severe diarrhea in infants and young children, the vaccine will have a tremendous impact on the health of children.

ROTAVIRUS VACCINE: SUMMARY AND CONCLUSIONS

Rotavirus causes high fever, vomiting, and diarrhea in infants and young children. Infection with rotavirus is so common and so severe that it causes one out of every 50 children in this country to be hospitalized with dehydration. We now have a rotavirus vaccine that is safe and protects against moderate-to-severe disease. The vaccine may be available by as early as 1998.

CHAPTER 29

LYME DISEASE

Jacob is 8 years old. After playing in the woods near his home in New Jersey, Jacob noticed a small tick on his leg. Jacob's mother knows that Lyme disease is carried by ticks in her area and wonders whether there is anything that can be done to prevent Jacob's getting infected.

Lyme disease is caused by a bacterium called *Borrelia burgdorferi* that is transmitted by the bite of a tick. The disease involves the joints, skin, nervous system, and heart and, if left untreated, can cause permanent damage to those tissues. At least 10,000 people each year develop Lyme disease in the United States.

A vaccine is currently being developed to prevent this disease.

What Is Lyme Disease?

Lyme disease was first recognized in 1975 when a number of children thought to have a form of childhood arthritis (inflammation of the joints) were seen in Lyme, Connecticut. The disease was called Lyme arthritis until it became clear that more than just the joints were involved.

Lyme disease is caused by a bacterium that is transmitted by the bite of a tick. Within a few days to a few weeks, the bacteria infect the skin that surrounds the tick bite and cause a red, circular rash, often with a pale center. The rash is accompanied by headache, fever, chills, achiness, and swollen glands.

Within a few weeks to a few months of the tick bite, the bacteria can also damage areas other than the skin. Joints such as the knee often become hot, tender, and swollen.

Excruciating headaches and neck pain occur when the bacteria infect the lining of the brain, causing meningitis. In addition, the bacteria can infect the brain itself (causing encephalitis) or individual nerves. For example, some people with Lyme disease are unable to move the muscles on one side of their face (called a facial palsy or Bell's palsy). This facial palsy is occasionally the only symptom of Lyme disease.

Lyme bacteria can also cause an irregular heart rate, or arrhythmia.

WHAT IS THE LYME VACCINE?

The bacterium that causes Lyme disease is coated by a number of proteins on the surface called outer surface proteins, or Osp. An immune response directed against these proteins appears to protect against disease.

One of the surface proteins (OspA) has been purified and used as a vaccine. Studies are currently being performed in adults to determine whether the vaccine is safe and effective.

Who gets Lyme disease?

Lyme disease has been reported in 47 states. However, children are most likely to get Lyme disease if they live in the Northeast (from Massachusetts to Maryland), the Midwest (Wisconsin and Minnesota), or the West (California and Oregon). Most disease occurs in June and July.

Lyme disease does not infect one particular age group; anyone at any age who is bitten by a tick is at risk.

Lyme Disease and Bites

Lyme disease is not only the most common tick-transmitted disease in the United States, but the most common insect-transmitted disease (including diseases spread by flies, mosquitoes, and fleas).

Why is it important to prevent Lyme disease?

There are a number of antibiotics that can be used to effectively treat Lyme disease. If someone is bitten by a tick and develops the early symptoms of Lyme disease, prompt recognition of the disease and appropriate treatment with antibiotics usually means that it will be mild.

Unfortunately, Lyme disease is sometimes not diagnosed in the early stages of infection and appropriate antibiotics are not prescribed. When this happens, the infection can spread to the joints and, in rare instances, to the nervous system or heart. Although appropriate antibiotics can cure Lyme disease even in the late stages, the best solution to the dilemma would be to have an effective vaccine.

When will the Lyme vaccine be available?

The Lyme vaccine may be available by 2000.

LYME VACCINE: SUMMARY AND CONCLUSIONS

Lyme disease can damage the joints, nervous system, and heart. Prompt recognition and treatment of this disease is sometimes necessary to avoid the possibility of permanent damage.

Unfortunately, early infection with Lyme disease may be difficult to recognize. The best way to avoid the damage caused by the disease is to prevent it with a vaccine. Although a promising candidate vaccine has been identified, it is unlikely that a Lyme vaccine will be available before 2000.

CHAPTER 30

RESPIRATORY SYNCYTIAL VIRUS ("THE VIRAL PNEUMONIA VACCINE")

Jenny is 18 months old. One day she developed a high fever and difficulty breathing. She was having so much trouble breathing that it was hard for her to hold down fluids. At the doctor's office, Jenny's mother was told that Jenny was wheezing. When the doctor got a chest X ray, he found that she also had pneumonia. The doctor told Jenny's mother that she would need to come into the hospital to receive oxygen therapy and intravenous (IV) fluids.

Is there anything that could have been done to prevent this?

Respiratory syncytial virus, or RSV, is the most common cause of severe lung disease in young children in this country. The first time a child is infected with RSV, he or she usually develops pneumonia or bronchiolitis (inflammation of the small breathing tubes, causing wheezing). Virtually every child will be infected by 2 years of age.

Every year about 100,000 children are hospitalized and 4,500 die from infections caused by RSV. That means that about one out of every 40 children born in this country will be hospitalized with RSV disease.

Although recent clinical trials have shown some promise, it is unlikely that an RSV vaccine will be available before 2005.

WHAT IS RESPIRATORY SYNCYTIAL VIRUS?

Respiratory syncytial virus infects the lungs of both children and adults. However, first-time infections with RSV usually occur by 2 years of age and are quite severe. More than 50 percent of children infected with the virus for the first time will develop either pneumonia or bronchiolitis, inflammation of the small breathing tubes of the lung. RSV also can occasionally cause croup (inflammation of the vocal cords and windpipe).

An infection with RSV begins with fever and a runny nose that lasts about three days. Children then develop difficulty breathing, rapid breathing, and a deepening cough. Some children will develop wheezing or croup, and many require hospitalization.

Children usually catch RSV from other children that are coughing or sneezing. The disease is highly contagious.

RSV and Ear Infections

Respiratory syncytial virus commonly causes ear infections. However, because RSV is a virus, it is not killed by antibiotics. Therefore, many children are given antibiotics unnecessarily for ear infections caused by RSV.

Why is it important to prevent RSV?

There is no drug that cures RSV infection. Therefore, an effective vaccine will probably be the best way to avoid the damage caused by this virus.

Is there anything other than waiting for a vaccine that I can do to prevent RSV in my children?

There is a medicine to prevent RSV infection called RespiGam®, which was recommended for use by the American Academy of Pediatrics in April of 1997. RespiGam® contains antibodies directed against RSV. Because children who were born premature (less than 32 weeks' gestation) and those who have lung disease from prematurity are at high risk of severe and occasionally fatal RSV infections, the American Academy of Pediatrics now recommends that RespiGam® be considered for use in these children. The medication is given intravenously once a month for the five months just prior to and during the winter season (when RSV is most likely to occur).

Although RespiGam® is of some value in preventing RSV infections, it is of no apparent value in treating the infections.

When can we expect to have a vaccine that prevents RSV?

There are no immediate prospects for an RSV vaccine.

Many approaches to develop a vaccine have been tried, using live weakened virus, killed virus, and purified viral proteins (see Chapter 3). Recent trials of an RSV vaccine in children with cystic fibrosis have shown some promise. Unfortunately, no vaccines have been proven clearly effective, and it is unlikely that one will be available before 2005.

RSV VACCINE:
SUMMARY AND CONCLUSIONS

RSV causes severe pneumonia and wheezing in infants and young children. Virtually every child will be infected with RSV within the first few years of life, and as many as one out of every 40 children born in this country will be hospitalized because of this infection. Unfortunately, it is unlikely that an RSV vaccine for use in all children will be available before 2005.

CHAPTER 31

AIDS

Elizabeth is 25 years old. She contracted HIV, the virus that causes AIDS, from a blood transfusion when she was in the hospital 15 years ago. Now she is pregnant and wonders whether there is a vaccine that she could be given to lessen her baby's risk of getting AIDS.

Will there soon be a vaccine to prevent AIDS?

The letters *AIDS* stand for *A*cquired *I*mmunodeficiency *S*yndrome. This disease is caused by the human immunodeficiency virus, or HIV. About 250,000 people in the United States have AIDS, and an estimated 5,000 of them are children.

Despite the enormous amount of time and money spent on understanding this disease, there are no immediate prospects for a vaccine. In this chapter we will discuss who gets AIDS, what the symptoms are, and why it has been so hard to develop an effective AIDS vaccine.

WHAT IS AIDS?

AIDS was first described in 1980. At that time, physicians in Los Angeles, New York, and San Francisco noticed that a number of young homosexual men either were infected by unusual microorganisms or had developed unusual cancers. In addition, the immune systems of these men were deficient; white blood cells (called lymphocytes) in the blood of these patients were either absent or few in number. Lymphocytes are important in helping the body fight infections.

Because these immunodeficiencies were occurring in previously healthy men, the disease was felt to have been recently acquired (as distinct from inherited or congenital). The syndrome was, therefore, called Acquired Immunodeficiency Syndrome, or AIDS.

In 1983, the disease was found to be caused by a virus that was later called human immunodeficiency virus, or HIV. The discovery of the virus that caused AIDS allowed scientists to develop a blood test. This blood test enabled doctors to tell whether someone was infected with HIV and whether blood that was used in transfusions was contaminated with the virus.

AIDS Is Spreading Across the World

AIDS was initially seen in North America, Western Europe, and sub-Saharan Africa. Now every continent on earth has people infected with HIV.

By the year 2000 it is expected that 30 to 40 million people (including 10 million children) will be infected with HIV and that 10 million people will have AIDS. In some parts of Africa, as many as 40 percent of young women are infected with HIV.

How can you tell if someone has AIDS?

Some people who are infected with HIV initially don't have any symptoms. Others will have fever, headache, swollen glands, and a sore throat that lasts for one or two weeks. These people are said to be HIV-infected.

About half of the people infected with HIV will develop more severe symptoms within ten years. Once they have developed severe symptoms, they are said to have AIDS. The symptoms that indicate that a patient may have AIDS are pneumonia caused by an unusual fungus (called *Pneumocystis carinii*), infection of the esophagus caused by a fungus (*Candida albicans*), or progressive loss of weight and energy (known as "wasting" syndrome).

Children who have AIDS get two additional diseases when they first develop severe symptoms. They may develop an unusual pneumonia of uncertain cause, as well as different kinds of recurrent bacterial infections.

How do children and adults get AIDS?

Children usually get AIDS by coming in contact with HIV-infected blood. Babies can become infected either while still in the womb or while passing through the birth canal of a mother with HIV. Also, children may have received blood transfusions from people who were infected with HIV.

Adults usually get AIDS by having sexual contact (either homosexual or heterosexual) with people who are infected with HIV. They can also get AIDS by receiving a blood transfusion from or sharing a syringe with someone who was infected with HIV.

The availability of a blood test for AIDS has virtually eliminated transfused blood as a source of HIV in the United States.

Why is it important to prevent AIDS?

There are several drugs available that help stop the growth of HIV in the body. These drugs both prolong the time from infection with HIV to development of AIDS and prolong the life of people who have AIDS after symptoms develop.

Unfortunately, because there is presently no cure for AIDS, the best hope to eliminate the disease will be to prevent it with an effective vaccine.

When will an AIDS vaccine be available?

Despite intensive worldwide efforts to understand the structure of HIV, how it causes disease, and how the body fights to prevent the disease, an effective vaccine is not at hand.

One of the reasons that it has been so hard to make an effective HIV vaccine is that the HIV strain that infects one person may be different from the strain that infects another. Researchers thus have tried to identify parts of the virus that are similar among many different strains and determine whether they would be suitable for a vaccine.

It is unlikely that there will be an effective HIV vaccine before 2005.

AIDS Vaccine:
Summary and Conclusions

About 250,000 people, including about 5,000 children, in the United States have AIDS. The disease is almost always fatal. Although the National Institutes of Health, as well as a number of pharmaceutical companies, have devoted considerable efforts to the development of an AIDS vaccine, there are no immediate prospects. It is unlikely that there will be a vaccine available to prevent AIDS before 2005.

VACCINES FOR TEENAGERS

Jon is 15 years old. His mother takes him to the doctor's office for a camp physical and finds out that he needs to get several vaccines. Jon's mother thought that he had already gotten all the vaccines he needed.

Are there vaccines specifically for teenagers?

Because teenagers don't get routine medical checkups, they aren't very good about getting the vaccines they need. Only 5 percent of 15-to-19-year-olds regularly visit their doctor. Most teenagers (and adults) wrongly assume that the vaccines they got as children were all that they needed for the rest of their lives.

The American Academy of Pediatrics now recommends a routine visit to the doctor for all children 11 to 12 years of age to provide the opportunity to receive four different vaccine preparations: varicella, hepatitis B, measles-mumps-rubella, and tetanus-diphtheria. For children 13 to 18 years of age, the same vaccines are of value. In this chapter we will discuss why it is important that teenagers get each of these vaccines.

VARICELLA (CHICKENPOX)

The varicella vaccine should be given to all teenagers who have not yet had chickenpox. Children who have managed to get to 13 years of age without getting chickenpox are at high risk of severe disease when they get varicella. This is because older teenagers and adults are more likely to develop pneumonia or encephalitis (inflammation of the brain) and are 15 times more likely to die from chickenpox than young children. For these reasons, the varicella vaccine was recently recommended for use in *all* children up to 18 years of age.

Recommendation by the American Academy of Pediatrics

The American Academy of Pediatrics recommends that all children between 11 and 12 years of age who have not previously had chickenpox receive a single dose of the varicella vaccine. In addition, all children between 13 and 18 years of age who have not had chickenpox should receive *two* doses of the varicella vaccine, given four to eight weeks apart.

One point about the varicella vaccine that is confusing to many parents is that the vaccine is recommended for teenagers who have "not previously been infected with varicella." But what should you do if you're not sure whether your child already had chickenpox? Some doctors recommend that if you're unsure, you should get a blood test to see if there is immunity to varicella (indicating that there was a previous chickenpox infection). However, we don't think this makes a lot of sense for two reasons. First, the blood test costs about the same as the vaccine. Second, adolescents who have already had chickenpox (and don't know it) won't be hurt by the vaccine. On the contrary, these teenagers will simply get a boost in their immunity to this virus.

For more information on the varicella vaccine, see Chapter 12.

HEPATITIS B

The hepatitis B vaccine was recommended for all newborns in 1991. But what about the many children and teenagers who did not receive the hepatitis B vaccine at birth—should they get the vaccine?

Recommendation by the American Academy of Pediatrics

The American Academy of Pediatrics recommends that all children 11 to 12 years of age receive the hepatitis B vaccine. The vaccine is given as a series of three shots. The second shot is given one to two months after the first shot, and the third shot is given four to six months after the first shot.

Although the hepatitis B vaccine is now recommended for all infants born in the United States, the groups most likely to catch the hepatitis B virus are teenagers and young adults. There are about 300,000 cases of hepatitis B virus infection in the United States every year, causing 10,000 hospitalizations and 400 deaths; as many as 24,000 people infected with the virus are teenagers. Therefore, it is very important to immunize children *before* they become teenagers. For this reason, the hepatitis B vaccine is recommended for all children at least by the time they are 11 to 12 years of age. In addition, we recommend that children between 13 and 18 years of age receive the vaccine.

For more information on the hepatitis B vaccine, see Chapter 11.

MEASLES-MUMPS-RUBELLA (MMR)

Severe outbreaks of measles occurred in high schools and on college campuses in the United States in the late 1980s—as many as 55,000 cases of measles were reported each year. Because of these outbreaks, the United States changed its policy on measles immunization in 1989. The recommendation now includes immunizing children 12 to 15 months of age *and* again at 4 to 6 years of age. But the most important part of this change is that *all* children should have at least *two* doses of measles vaccine by the time they enter high school. This means that some children will get the second dose of the vaccine between 11 and 12 years of age.

Recommendation by the American Academy of Pediatrics

The American Academy of Pediatrics recommends that all children who have not received two doses of MMR vaccine receive a second dose, preferably at 11 to 12 years of age. Those who have not received two doses by age 18 should receive the second dose at that time.

Why did these measles outbreaks occur? Most of the teenagers and young adults infected with measles during these outbreaks had *never* received the measles vaccine; some had received the vaccine but didn't develop immunity. The requirement for a second dose of the vaccine gives many children their first chance to get it. In addition, for some children the second dose of vaccine gives them a chance to acquire the immunity that they failed to get after the first dose. In any case, the new recommendation is working. In 1990 there were about 28,000 cases of measles reported to the Centers for Disease Control and Prevention; in 1995, there were only 300.

The second dose of mumps and rubella vaccines is given along with the measles vaccine for the reasons cited above; for many children, this is their first chance to receive the vaccines, and for others it is a chance to develop the immunity they did not receive from the first dose.

For more information on the measles-mumps-rubella vaccine, see Chapter 10.

TETANUS–DIPHTHERIA

Why do we need to boost the tetanus vaccine every ten years? The main reason is that immunity to tetanus fades over time. Also, teenagers and adults are always at risk for "tetanus-prone" injuries. These injuries include any puncture wounds contaminated with soil (for example, nails penetrating through sneakers). Indeed, most deaths associated with tetanus occur in adults.

Recommendation by the American Academy of Pediatrics

The American Academy of Pediatrics recommends that children receive the tetanus and diphtheria vaccines (in a preparation called Td) every ten years, beginning at 11 to 12 years of age.

The diphtheria vaccine is given along with the tetanus vaccine because, as with the tetanus vaccine, immunity to the diphtheria vaccine fades over time. In addition, an epidemic of diphtheria is now raging in the former Soviet Union. More than 120,000 cases, causing 4,000 deaths, occurred between 1990 and 1995. Most of those infected were not vaccinated, and most cases occurred in adults.

Diphtheria is still around in the United States. Forty-one cases and four deaths were reported between 1980 and 1995. For more information, see Chapter 7.

CHAPTER 33

VACCINES FOR ADULTS (INCLUDING GRANDPARENTS)

Wendy is 40 years old. She takes her 15-year-old son to the doctor and finds out that he needs both the varicella and the hepatitis B vaccines. She is pretty sure that she has never had either chickenpox or hepatitis. Should she get these vaccines too?

Are there any other vaccines that you need when you are an adult?

Although it may be hard to believe, every year in the United States *100 times* more adults die from vaccine-preventable diseases than children. How is this possible? First, pneumonia, caused by influenza and pneumococcus, kills 50,000 adults annually. Second, hepatitis B virus infects about 300,000 adults and kills 5,000. And third, although rare, almost all deaths caused by tetanus and diphtheria occur in adults. So

199

whereas about 500 children die every year from diseases that are clearly preventable by vaccines, between 50,000 to 70,000 adults die from these same diseases.

Although getting vaccines is not considered by many as an adult thing to do, all adults should consider the following vaccinations for themselves.

I am 45 years old and haven't had any shots for years. What vaccines do I need?

There are four vaccines that should be considered for use in all adults: hepatitis B, varicella, measles, and diphtheria-tetanus. Each of these vaccines is discussed below.

All adults who have had neither a hepatitis B virus infection nor the hepatitis B vaccine should get vaccinated (see Chapter 11). The vaccine is given as a series of three shots over a six-month period.

All adults who have not had a varicella infection should be vaccinated. The vaccine is given as a series of two shots over a four-to-eight-week period. If one is unsure about previous infection, we recommend receiving the vaccine (see Chapter 12 for more details).

All adults born after 1956 (and, therefore, unlikely to have been naturally infected with measles virus) should receive two doses of the measles vaccine if they have been neither previously immunized nor infected with the virus. The vaccine should be given in the preparation called MMR, which also includes the mumps and rubella vaccines. The addition of mumps and rubella vaccines will allow for either a first-time immunization to those viruses or a boost in immunity (see Chapter 10 for more details).

Adults should receive booster doses of the tetanus and diphtheria vaccines every ten years, starting at 20 to 25 years of age. The vaccine is given in a preparation called Td (see Chapter 7 for more details).

Vaccines for All Adults

All adults who haven't been previously infected should be immunized with varicella, hepatitis B, tetanus-diphtheria, and measles.

I am 68 years old. What vaccines do I need?

In addition to the four listed above, there are two more vaccines that should be considered for people over 65 years of age: influenza and pneumococcus.

Healthy adults over 65 years of age are at high risk of developing severe and occasionally fatal infections with influenza and pneumococcus, as compared with younger adults. For this reason, *all* adults older than 65 are recommended to receive both the pneumococcal and influenza vaccines (see Chapters 16 and 17 for more details).

Which adults need the influenza vaccine?

All adults over 65 years of age are at risk of severe pneumonia caused by influenza and should receive the influenza vaccine every year. About 90 percent of deaths from influenza occur among people older than 65 years. In addition, those at high risk of coming in contact with the influenza virus should be vaccinated. This group includes doctors, nurses, and other health care workers. Even pregnant health care workers can be vaccinated, because the vaccine doesn't harm the fetus.

There are other groups of adults that are also at high risk for severe pneumonia when they get an influenza infection. For example, there is recent evidence that normal, healthy women in their third trimester of pregnancy may have a more serious case of influenza. For this reason, the Centers for Disease Control and Prevention now ask doctors to consider the influenza vaccine for all pregnant women whose third trimester falls within the influenza season (December to March). In addition, the vaccine should be used in people with long-standing heart, kidney, or lung disease (including asthma) and those with diabetes.

It should be noted that even healthy children and adults living in the same home as people at high risk of severe influenza disease should be immunized.

Which adults need the pneumococcal vaccine?

All adults over 65 years of age are at high risk of severe pneumonia caused by the pneumococcus bacteria and should, therefore, receive the pneumococcal vaccine. In addition, all adults with long-standing heart or lung disease, liver disease, alcoholism, diabetes, or cancer should receive the vaccine.

Unfortunately, people who need the pneumococcal vaccine often don't receive it. Only 15 percent of people over 65 years of age get the vaccine, and only 8 percent of those between 50 and 64 years of age at high risk for severe disease get vaccinated.

My child is in a day care center. Are there vaccines that employees of the center should get?

It is especially important for day care center workers to be immunized with the following vaccines: measles-mumps-rubella, tetanus-diphtheria, varicella, hepatitis B, influenza, and hepatitis A.

The hepatitis A virus is a common cause of infection in day care centers and like, chickenpox, is much more severe in adults than children. Therefore, all adults who work in day care centers should be immunized with the hepatitis A vaccine. This vaccine is given as a series of two shots over a six-month period (see Chapter 21).

CONCLUSION: MAKING DECISIONS ABOUT VACCINES

In April of 1997, a 7-year-old boy was seen in the emergency room of The Children's Hospital of Philadelphia. The boy's mother said that the child had for several days had chickenpox. He had hundreds of blisters covering him from head to toe and a high fever. But it wasn't the chickenpox that worried her. Centered on one of the blisters, on the inside of his left arm, was a painful, swollen, purple area covering his entire upper arm as well as the left side of his chest. Because of the swelling on his chest, he was having difficulty breathing.

The doctors in the emergency room admitted the boy to the hospital and eventually made the diagnosis. The swelling was due to a poison, or toxin, produced by a bacterium called Group A b-hemolytic streptococcus (often referred to in the media as the "flesh-eating" bacterium). The child was given antibiotics and, although it was touch-and-go for about two weeks, survived.

The irony of this story is that the boy had visited his doctor three weeks before he got chickenpox. The doctor had told the boy's mother that there was a new vaccine available to prevent chickenpox and that the decision of whether to give him the varicella vaccine was up to her. She interpreted the doctor's lukewarm recommendation as ambivalence and decided not to give the vaccine to her son.

Unfortunately, the mother didn't have all the facts she needed to make her decision. She didn't know that every year 9,000 children, most of them previously healthy, are hospitalized with chickenpox infections. She didn't know that the varicella vaccine had been tested in this and other countries for about 20 years, and that immunity didn't fade. Nor did she know that the number of cases of children with "flesh-eating" bacteria because of chickenpox was on the rise. If she had known these facts, her decision might have been different.

In this book we have tried to include the information that parents need to make decisions about vaccines. We have also chosen to explain in a simple manner some fairly complex issues regarding the science, immunology, and biology of vaccines. We did this because we wanted parents to understand not only the facts, but also the concepts behind vaccines. Now when parents are asked to participate in decisions about vaccines, we have no doubt that they will be compelling advocates for their children's health.

BIBLIOGRAPHY

GENERAL

Plotkin, S. A., and Mortimer, E. A. *Vaccines.* 2nd ed. Philadelphia: W. B. Saunders and Co., 1994.

Parents' Guide to Childhood Immunization. Centers for Disease Control and Prevention, U.S. Department of Health and Human Services.

Peter, G., ed. *1997 Red Book: Report of Committee on Infectious Diseases.* 24th ed. Elk Grove Village, IL: American Academy of Pediatrics, 1997.

Six Common Misconceptions About Vaccination. Centers for Disease Control and Prevention, U.S. Department of Health and Human Services.

Atkinson, W., Furphy, L., Gantt, J., et al., eds. *Epidemiology and Prevention of Vaccine-Preventable Diseases.* 3rd ed. Centers for Disease Control and Prevention, U.S. Department of Health and Human Services, 1996.

Your Child's Best Shot: A Parent's Guide to Vaccination. Canadian Pediatric Society, Ottawa, Ontario.

Mandell, G. L., Bennett, J. E., and Dolin, R., eds. *Principles and Practice of Infectious Diseases.* 4th ed. New York: Churchill Livingstone, 1995.

Guide to Contraindications to Childhood Vaccinations. Centers for Disease Control and Prevention, U.S. Department of Health and Human Services.

Feigin, R. D., and Cherry, J. D., ed. *Textbook of Pediatric Infectious Diseases.* 3rd ed. Philadelphia: W. B. Saunders and Co., 1992.

On the Internet

Information about vaccines from the Centers for Disease Control and Prevention can be found at www.cdc/gov/nip

HOW ARE VACCINES MADE?

The story of mumps

Buynak, E. B., and Hilleman, M. R. "Live attenuated mumps virus vaccine. I. Vaccine development." *Proceedings of the Society of Experimental Biology and Medicine,* vol. 123, pp. 768–775, 1966.

Hilleman, M. R., Buynak, E. B., Weibel, R. E., and Stokes, J., Jr. "Live, attenuated mumps-virus vaccine." *The New England Journal of Medicine,* vol. 278, pp. 227–232, 1968.

Pagano, J. S., Levine, R. H., Sugg, W. C., and Finger, J. A. "Clinical trial of new attenuated mumps virus vaccine (Jeryl Lynn Strain): preliminary report." *Progress in Immunobiologic Standardization.* vol. 3, pp. 196–202, New York: Karger, Basel, 1969.

"Mumps Vaccine: Recommendation of the Public Health Service Advisory Committee on Immunization Practices." *Morbidity and Mortality Weekly Report,* vol. 26, pp. 393–394, 1977.

Interview with Maurice Hilleman on December 3, 1996.

The Cutter incident

Nathanson, N., and Langmuir, A. D. "The Cutter incident: poliomyelitis following formaldehyde-inactivated poliovirus vaccination in the United States during the spring of 1955." I. Background. *American Journal of Hygiene,* vol. 78, pp. 16–28, 1963.

Nathanson, N., and Langmuir, A. D. "The Cutter incident: poliomyelitis following formaldehyde-inactivated poliovirus vaccination in the United States during the spring of 1955." II. Relationship of poliomyelitis to Cutter vaccine. *American Journal of Hygiene,* vol. 78, pp. 16–28, 1963.

Hinman, A. R., and Thacker, S. B. Invited commentary on "The Cutter incident": poliomyelitis following formaldehyde-inactivated poliovirus vaccination in the United States during the spring of 1955. II. Relationship of poliomyelitis to Cutter vaccine. *American Journal of Epidemiology,* vol. 142, pp. 107–108, 1995.

The story of the RSV vaccine

Kapikian, A. Z., Mitchell, R. H., Chanock, R. M., et al. "An epide-miologic study of altered clinical reactivity to respiratory syncytial (RS) virus infection in children previously vaccinated with inactivated RS virus vaccine." *American Journal of Epidemiology,* vol. 89, pp. 405–421, 1969.

Kim, H. W., Canchola, J. G., Brandt, C. D., et al. "Respiratory syncytial virus disease in infants despite prior administration of antigen inactivated vaccine." *American Journal of Epidemiology,* vol. 89, pp. 422–434, 1969.

Chin, J., Magoffin, R. L., Shearer, L. A., et al. "Field evaluation of a respiratory syncytial vaccine and a trivalent parainfluenza virus vaccine in a pediatric population." *American Journal of Epidemi-ology,* vol. 89, pp. 449–463, 1969.

Fulginiti, V. A., Eller, J. J., Sieber, O. F., et al. "Respiratory virus immunization. I. A field trial of two inactivated respiratory virus vaccines; an aqueous trivalent parainfluenza virus vaccine and an alum-precipitated respiratory syncytial virus vaccine." *American Journal of Epidemiology,* vol. 89, pp. 435–448, 1969.

Piedra, P. A., Hiatt, P. W., Grace, S., et al. "Safety and efficacy of PFP-2 vaccine during respiratory syncytial virus season in children with cystic fibrosis." Presented at the 36th Interscience Conference on Antimicrobial Agents and Chemotherapy, New Orleans. September 15–18, 1996. Abstract H50.

ARE VACCINES SAFE?

Budnick, L. D., and Ross, D. A. "Bathtub-related drownings in the United States, 1979–1981." *American Journal of Public Health,* vol. 75, pp. 630–633, 1985.

Baker, S. P. *The Injury Fact Book.* Lexington, MA: Lexington Books, 1984.

Duclos, P. J., and Sanderson, L. M. "An epidemiological description of lightning-related deaths in the United States." *International Journal of Epidemiology,* vol. 19, pp. 673–679, 1990.

"Update: Vaccine side effects, adverse reactions, contraindications, and precautions." *Morbidity and Mortality Weekly Report,* vol. 45, September 6, 1996.

Howson, C. P., Howe, C. J., Fineberg, H. V., eds. *Adverse Effects of Pertussis and Rubella Vaccines.* Washington, D.C.: National Academy Press, 1991.

Stratton, K. R., Howe, C. J., Johnston, R. B. Jr., eds. *Adverse Events Associated with Childhood Vaccines: Evidence Bearing on Causality.* Washington, D.C.: National Academy Press, 1994.

Ross, J. F. "Risk: Where do real dangers lie?" *Smithsonian,* November 1995.

Dingle, J. G., Badger, G. F., Jordan, W. S. *Illness in the Home: A Study of 25,000 Illnesses in a Group of Cleveland Families.* Cleveland: The Press of Western Reserve University, 1964.

WHO RECOMMENDS VACCINES?

Title 28, Part III, Chapter 23, Subchapter C of the Commonwealth of Pennsylvania's School Health Immunization Legislation.

WHEN DO CHILDREN GET VACCINES?

"Recommended childhood immunization schedule—United States, January–December 1997." *Pediatrics,* vol. 99, pp. 136–138, 1997.

DTaP

"Update: Vaccine side effects, adverse reactions, contraindications, and precautions." *Morbidity and Mortality Weekly Report,* vol. 45, September 6, 1996.

Howson, C. P., and Fineberg, H. V. "Adverse events following pertussis and rubella vaccines: summary of a report of the Institute of Medicine." *Journal of the American Medical Association,* vol. 267, pp. 392–396, 1992.

Wortis, N., Strebel, P. M., Wharton, M., et al. "Pertussis deaths: report of 23 cases in the United States, 1992–1993." *Pediatrics,* vol. 97, pp. 607–612, 1996.

Greco, D., Salmaso, S., Mastrantonio, P., et al. "A controlled trial of two acellular vaccines and one whole-cell vaccine against pertussis." *The New England Journal of Medicine,* vol. 334, pp. 341–348, 1996.

Griffin, M. R., Ray, W. A., Livengood, J. R., et al. "Risk of sudden infant death syndrome after immunization with the diphtheria-tetanus-pertussis vaccine." *The New England Journal of Medicine,* vol. 319, pp. 618–623, 1988.

Rock, A. "The lethal dangers of the billion-dollar vaccine business." *Money,* pp. 148–164, December 1996.

Committee on Infectious Diseases of the American Academy of Pediatrics. "Acellular pertussis vaccine: recommendations for use as the initial series in infants and children." *Pediatrics,* vol. 99, pp. 282–288, 1997.

POLIO

Black, K. *In the Shadow of Polio: A Personal and Social History.* Boston: Addison-Wesley Publishing Co., 1996.

Judelsohn, R. "Changing the US polio immunization schedule would be bad public health policy." *Pediatrics,* vol. 98, pp. 115–116, 1996.

Katz, S. "Poliovirus policy—time for a change." *Pediatrics,* vol. 98, pp. 116–117, 1996.

Plotkin, S. A. "Inactivated polio vaccine for the United States: a missed vaccination opportunity." *Pediatric Infectious Diseases Journal,* vol. 14, pp. 835–839, 1995.

Nkowane, B. M., Wassilak, S. G. F., Orenstein, W. A., et al. "Vaccine-associated paralytic poliomyelitis." *Journal of the American Medical Association,* vol. 257, pp. 1335–1340, 1987.

Paradiso, P. R. "The future of polio immunization in the United States: are we ready for a change?" *Pediatric Infectious Disease Journal,* vol. 15, pp. 645–649, 1996.

Faden, H., Modlin, J. F., Thoms, M. L., et al. "Comparative evaluation of immunization with live attenuated and enhanced-potency inactivated trivalent poliovirus vaccines in childhood: systemic and local immune responses." *The Journal of Infectious Diseases,* vol. 162, pp. 1291–1297, 1990.

HIB

"Recommendations for use of Haemophilus b conjugate vaccines and a combined Diphtheria, Tetanus, Pertussis, and Haemophilus b vaccine." *Morbidity and Mortality Weekly Report,* vol. 42, September 17, 1993.

MMR

Measles

"Update: Vaccine side effects, adverse reactions, contraindications, and precautions." *Morbidity and Mortality Weekly Report,* vol. 45, September 6, 1996.

Wicks, S. *History of Medicine in New Jersey.* Newark, NJ: M. R. Dennis and Co., 1879.

James, J. M., Burks, A. W., Robertson, P. K., and Sampson, H. A. "Safe administration of the measles vaccine to children allergic to eggs." *The New England Journal of Medicine,* vol. 332, pp. 1262–1266, 1995.

Watson, J. C., Pearson, J. A., Markowitz, L. E., et al. "An evaluation of measles revaccination among school-entry aged children." *Pediatrics,* vol. 97, pp. 613–618, 1996.

Davis, S. F., Strebel, P. M., Atkinson, W. L., et al. "Reporting efficiency during a measles outbreak in New York City, 1991." *American Journal of Public Health,* vol. 83, pp. 1011–1015, 1993.

Mumps

"Update: Vaccine side effects, adverse reactions, contraindications, and precautions." *Morbidity and Mortality Weekly Report,* vol. 45, September 6, 1996.

Hilleman, M. R. "Past, present and future of measles, mumps, and rubella virus vaccines." *Pediatrics,* vol. 90, pp. 149–153, 1992.

Rubella

Howson, C. P., and Fineberg, H. V. "The ricochet of magic bullets: summary of the Institute of Medicine report, Adverse effects of pertussis and rubella vaccines." *Pediatrics,* vol. 89, pp. 318–324, 1992.

Fulginiti, V. A. "How safe are the pertussis and rubella vaccines? A commentary on the Institute of Medicine report." *Pediatrics,* vol. 89, pp. 334–336, 1992.

Gregg, N. M. "Congenital cataract following German measles in the mother." *Transactions of the Ophthalmologic Society of Australia,* vol. 3, pp. 35–46, 1941.

HEPATITIS B

Szmuness, W., Stevens, C. E., Harley, E. J., et al. "Hepatitis B vaccine: demonstration of efficacy in a controlled clinical trial in a high-risk population in the United States." *The New England Journal of Medicine,* vol. 303, pp. 833–841, 1980.

Dienstag, J. L. "Toward the control of hepatitis B." *The New England Journal of Medicine,* vol. 303, pp. 875–876, 1980.

Mulley, A. G., Silverstein, M. D., and Dienstag, J. L. "Indications for use of hepatitis B vaccine, based on cost-effectiveness analysis." *The New England Journal of Medicine,* vol. 307, pp. 644–652, 1982.

"Universal hepatitis B immunization." *Pediatrics,* vol. 89, pp. 795–800, 1992.

"Hepatitis B virus: a comprehensive strategy for eliminating transmission in the United States through universal childhood vaccination." Recommendations of the Immunization Practices Advisory Committee (ACIP). *Morbidity and Mortality Weekly Report,* vol. 40, November 22, 1991.

"Update: Vaccine side effects, adverse reactions, contraindications, and precautions." *Morbidity and Mortality Weekly Report,* vol. 45, September 6, 1996.

Muraskin, W. "The war against hepatitis B: a history of the international task force on hepatitis B immunization." Philadelphia: University of Pennsylvania Press, 1995.

VARICELLA

Fleisher, G., Henry, W., McSorley, M., et al. "Life-threatening complications of varicella." *American Journal of Diseases in Children,* vol. 135, pp. 896–899, 1981.

Pastuszak, A. L., Levy, M., Schick, B., et al. "Outcome after maternal varicella infection in the first 20 weeks of pregnancy." *The New England Journal of Medicine,* vol. 330, pp. 901–905, 1994.

Doctor, A., Harper, M. B., and Fleisher, G. R. "Group A B-hemolytic streptococcal bacteremia: historical overview, changing incidence, and recent association with varicella." *Pediatrics,* vol. 96, pp. 428–433, 1995.

Weibel, R. E., Neff, B. J., Kuter, B. J., et al. "Live, attenuated varicella virus vaccine: efficacy trial in healthy children." *The New England Journal of Medicine,* vol. 310, pp. 1409–1415, 1984.

"Recommendations for the use of live attenuated varicella vaccine." *Pediatrics,* vol. 95, pp. 791–796, 1995.

Plotkin, S. A. "Varicella vaccine." *Pediatrics,* vol. 97, pp. 251–253, 1996.

Asano, Y., Suga, S., Yoshikawa, T., et al. "Experience and reason: twenty-year follow-up of protective immunity of the Oka strain live varicella vaccine." *Pediatrics,* vol. 94, pp. 524–526, 1994.

Hardy, I., Gershon, A. A., Steinberg, S. P., et al. "The incidence of zoster after immunization with live attenuated varicella vaccine: a study in children with leukemia." *The New England Journal of Medicine,* vol. 325, pp. 1545–1550, 1991.

PRACTICAL TIPS ABOUT VACCINES

Peter, G., ed. *1997 Red Book: Report of the Committee on Infectious Diseases.* 24th ed. Elk Grove Village, IL: American Academy of Pediatrics, 1997.

French, G. M., Painter, E. C. Coury, D. L. "Blowing away shot pain: a technique for pain management during immunization." *Pediatrics,* vol. 93, pp. 384–388, 1994.

THE GREAT VACCINE MYTHS

"Vaccination: the issue of our times." In *Mothering: The Magazine of Natural Family Living,* no. 79, pp. 26–80, Summer 1996.

Curtis, T. "The Origin of AIDS: a startling new theory attempts to answer the question 'Was it an act of God or an act of man?'", *Rolling Stone,* March 19, 1992.

Khan, A. S., Shahabuddin, M., Bryan, T., et al. "Analysis of live, oral poliovirus vaccine monopools for human immunodeficiency virus type 1 and simian immunodeficiency virus." *The Journal of Infectious Diseases,* vol. 174, pp. 1185–1190, 1996.

Garrett, A. J., Dunham, A., Wood, D. J. "Retroviruses and polio vaccines." *The Lancet,* pp. 932–933, October 9, 1993.

Wechsler, P. "A Shot in the Dark." *New York,* pp. 39–85, November 11, 1996.

Carbone, M., Rizzo, P., Procopic, A., et al. "SV40-like sequences in human bone tumors." *Oncogene,* vol. 13, pp. 527–535, 1996.

Carbone, M., Pass, H. I., Rizzo, P., et al. "Simian virus 40-like DNA sequences in human pleural mesothelioma." *Oncogene,* vol. 9, pp. 1781–1790, 1994.

Rock, A. "The lethal dangers of the billion-dollar vaccine business." *Money,* pp. 148–164, December 1996.

Cohn, M., Langman, R. E. "The Protecton: The unit of humoral immunity selected by evolution." *Immunological Reviews,* vol. 115, pp. 11–147, 1990.

Miller, N. Z. *Vaccines: Are They Really Safe and Effective?* Santa Fe, NM: New Atlantean Press, 1996.

Neustaedter, R. *The Vaccine Guide: Making an Informed Choice.* Berkeley, CA: North Atlantic Books, 1996.

RABIES

Fishbein, D. B., and Robinson, L. E. "Rabies." *The New England Journal of Medicine,* vol. 329, pp. 1632–1638, 1993.

de Kruif, P. *Microbe Hunters.* New York: Harcourt, Brace and Co., 1926.

INFLUENZA

"Prevention and control of influenza: recommendations of the Advisory Committee on Immunization Practices (ACIP)." *Morbidity and Mortality Weekly Report,* vol. 45, May 3, 1996.

Murphy, K. R., and Strunk, R. C. "Safe administration of influenza vaccine in asthmatic children hypersensitive to egg proteins." *The Journal of Pediatrics,* vol. 106, pp. 931–933, 1985.

Wade, N. "1976 swine flu campaign faulted yet principals would do it again." *Science,* vol. 202, pp. 849–852, 1978.

Asbury, A. K. "The swine flu incident revisited." *Annals of Neurology,* vol. 16, pp. 513–514, 1984.

Beghi, E., Kurland, L. T., Mulder, D. W., and Wiederholt, W. C. "Guillain-Barré syndrome: clinicoepidemiologic features and effect of influenza vaccine." *Archives of Neurology,* vol. 42, pp. 1053–1057, 1985.

Safranek, T. J., Lawrence, D. N., Kurland, L. T., et al. "Reassessment of the association between Guillain-Barré syndrome and receipt of swine influenza vaccine in 1976–1977: results of a two-state study." *American Journal of Epidemiology,* vol. 133, pp. 940–951, 1991.

Hoehling, A. A. *The Great Epidemic.* Boston: Little Brown and Co., 1961.

PNEUMOCOCCUS

"Immunization Practices Advisory Committee: Pneumococcal polysaccharide vaccine." *Morbidity and Mortality Weekly Report,* vol. 38, p. 64, 1989.

Sims, R. V. "Pneumococcal vaccine: a continuing controversy." *Hospital Practice,* April 30, 1992.

TUBERCULOSIS

Bates, J. H., Stead, W. W. "The history of tuberculosis as a global epidemic." *Medical Clinics of North America,* vol. 77, pp. 1205–1217, 1993.

Houk, V. H., Kent, D. C., Baker, J. H., et al. "The Byrd study: in-depth analysis of a micro-outbreak of tuberculosis in a closed environment." *Archives of Environmental Health,* vol. 16, pp. 4–6, 1968.

Stead, W. W. "Tuberculosis among elderly persons: an outbreak in a nursing home." *Annals of Internal Medicine,* vol. 94, pp. 606–610, 1981.

"The role of BCG vaccine in the prevention and control of tuberculosis in the United States: a joint statement by the Advisory Council for the Elimination of Tuberculosis and the Advisory Committee on Immunization Practices." *Morbidity and Mortality Weekly Report,* vol. 45, April 26, 1996.

Grange, J. M., Gibson, J., Osborn, T. W., et al. "What is BCG?" *Tubercle,* vol. 64, pp. 129–139, 1983.

SOURCES OF INFORMATION ABOUT VACCINES FOR TRAVELERS

Wade, B. "Finding out about vaccines." *New York Times,* November 24, 1996.

"Health Information for International Travel 1996–97." U.S. Department of Health and Human Services. Centers for Disease Control and Prevention. National Center for Infectious Diseases. Atlanta, Georgia.

HEPATITIS A

"Licensure of inactivated hepatitis A vaccine and recommendations for use among international travelers." *Morbidity and Mortality Weekly Report,* vol. 44, pp. 559–560, 1995.

Margolis, H. S., and Alter, M. J. "Will hepatitis A become a vaccine-preventable disease?" *Annals of Internal Medicine,* vol. 122, pp. 464–465, 1995.

CHOLERA

"Recommendation of the Immunization Practices Advisory Committee (ACIP): Cholera vaccine." *Morbidity and Mortality Weekly Report,* vol. 37, pp. 617–624, 1988.

Mann, T. *Death in Venice.* New York: Alfred A. Knopf, 1930.

Typhoid

"Typhoid immunization: recommendations of the Advisory Committee on Immunization Practices (ACIP)." *Morbidity and Mortality Weekly Report,* vol. 43, December 9, 1994.

Japanese Encephalitis Virus

"Inactivated Japanese encephalitis virus vaccine: recommendations of the Advisory Committee on Immunization Practices (ACIP)." *Morbidity and Mortality Weekly Report,* vol. 42, January 8, 1993.

RSV

Committee on Infectious Diseases, Committee on Fetus and Newborn, American Academy of Pediatrics. "Respiratory syncytial virus immune globulin intravenous: indications for use." *Pediatrics,* vol. 99, pp. 645–650, 1997.

Rodriguez, W. J., W. C. Gruber, R. C. Welliver, et al. "Respiratory syncytial virus (RSV) immune globulin intravenous therapy for RSV lower respiratory tract infection in infants and young children at high risk for severe RSV infections." *Pediatrics,* vol. 99, pp. 454–461, 1997.

Piedra, P. A., Hiatt, P. W., Grace, S., et al. "Safety and efficacy of PFP-2 vaccine during respiratory syncytial virus season in children with cystic fibrosis." Presented at the 36th Interscience Conference on Antimicrobial Agents and Chemotherapy, New Orleans. September 15–18, 1996. Abstract H50.

Vaccines for Adults

"Update on adult immunization: recommendations of the Immunization Practices Advisory Subcommittee (ACIP)". *Morbidity and Mortality Weekly Report,* vol. 40, November 15, 1991.

Gardner, P., and Schaffner, W. "Immunization of adults." *The New England Journal of Medicine,* vol. 328, pp. 1252–1258, 1993.

ABOUT THE AUTHORS

PAUL A. OFFIT

Dr. Offit is chief of the Section of Infectious Diseases at the Children's Hospital of Philadelphia and an Associate Professor of Pediatrics at the University of Pennsylvania School of Medicine. He is the recipient of a number of awards including the J. Edmund Bradley Prize for Excellence in Pediatrics, the Young Investigator Award in Vaccine Development, and the University of Pennsylvania Research Foundation Award. He is an internationally recognized expert in the fields of immunology and virology.

LOUIS M. BELL

Dr. Bell is an attending physician in the sections of Infectious Diseases and Emergency Medicine at the Children's Hospital of Philadelphia and an Associate Professor of Pediatrics at The University of Pennsylvania School of Medicine. He is the recipient of many awards including an outstanding achievement award in early childhood immunization presented by the U.S. Secretary of Health and Human Services and the Dean's Award from the University of Pennsylvania School of Medicine for excellence in clinical teaching. He is also the recipient of a grant from the Centers for Disease Control and Prevention to enhance preschool immunizations and served as co-chair of the West Philadelphia Immunization Project.

INDEX

for children living with
someone with weakened
immunity, 92–93
combination, 173–75
and fear of shots, 91–92
how they work, 5–8
illness and, 93
making decisions about, 203–4
making of, 9–17
missed, 95
myths about. *See* Myths about
vaccines
need for, 3–4
practical tips about, 91–96
pregnancy and. *See* Pregnancy
for premature babies, 95
recommended, 26–27, 28, 140
required, 27–28, 140
right to refuse, public health
vs., 28–29
safety of. *See* Safety of vaccines
severe reactions to, 92
simultaneous, 95
steroids and, 93–94
for teenagers. *See* Teenagers,
vaccines for
travel and. *See* Travel, vaccines
for
weakened viruses and bacteria
in, 7, 8, 9–10, 11
when to get, 33–35
who should not get, 92
Varicella vaccine. *See* Chickenpox
vaccine
Viral pneumonia vaccine (RSV
vaccine), 17, 185–88
Viruses, 7–8
in making of vaccines, 7, 8,
9–10, 11

W–Z

Water, traveler's diarrhea and,
164–66
Whooping cough. *See* Pertussis
Yellow fever, 139, 155, 156–57
Yellow fever vaccine, 94, 139,
155–57
safety of, 156